Pearls for Leaders

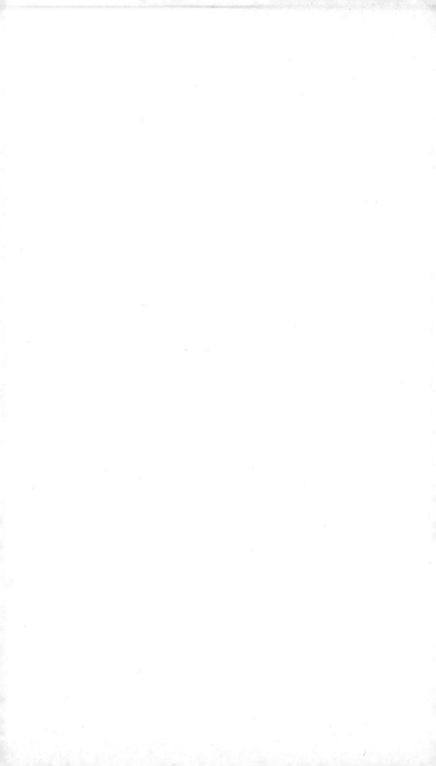

Pearls for Leaders in Academic Medicine

By

Emery A. Wilson, MD
Jay A. Perman, MD
D. Kay Clawson, MD

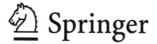 Springer

Emery A. Wilson, MD
University of Kentucky
College of Medicine
Lexington, KY
USA
ewilson@email.uky.edu

Jay A. Perman, MD
University of Kentucky
College of Medicine
Lexington, KY
USA
jperman@uky.edu

D. Kay Clawson, MD
University of Kentucky
College of Medicine
Lexington, KY
USA
dkcjd@insightbb.com

ISBN: 978-0-387-77113-7   e-ISBN: 978-0-387-77114-4
DOI: 10.1007/978-0-387-77114-4

Library of Congress Control Number: 2008922191

Printed on acid-free paper

9 8 7 6 5 4 3 2 1

springer.com

Preface

This book, like its predecessor, *The Medical School Dean: Reflections and Directions,* is written out of concern for developing leaders of academic medicine. While the strength of any medical school is its faculty and students, the preparation and stability of the leadership is critical to its success in its various missions.

Recently, the leaders of the Association of American Medical Colleges became concerned when it learned that the average term in office for medical school deans was less than four years in duration. There was actually a bimodal distribution to the longevity of deans, with some serving only a year or two while others had been in place for several years. The Leadership Committee was established to support deans and to improve their longevity in the position. Several factors were found to decrease the time in the position:

- **The search process may not have identified the right person.**
- **Personal, communication, or management skills were lacking.**
- **The new dean may have been more interested in furthering his/her own career rather than the careers of the faculty.**
- **The dean did not have the respect of the university president or other superior.**

The same factors may be operating in the success or failure of other leaders of academic medicine, such as chairs, center directors, and divisions chiefs. As a consequence, the information in this book is directed to leaders and potential leaders at all levels of academic medicine.

Although a new administrator usually has a "honeymoon period" for a couple of years, that sometimes can lead to a level of false confidence. Faculty acceptance of decisions early in one's career can cause the administrator to want to implement major change, which causes his/her downfall and the beginning of another flawed search.

The search process for medical school leaders is an ill-defined and cumbersome process. Candidates from within the school are often overlooked in favor of outside candidates who may have burgeoning curricula vitae and who are perceived to bring new ideas to the institution. Great curricula vitae often take precedence over great leaders. Because of the expense of the search process and because great leaders can come from within, medical schools should put more emphasis on succession planning at all administrative levels. However, medical schools are not usually concerned about succession plans, so many administrators come to the positions ill-prepared. Many are not familiar with the organizational structure of the school or the budget process, and they certainly are not prepared for the confrontations encountered when a decision is made.

Any decision of substance seems to make someone angry. Chairs and faculty members who were friends and colleagues are no longer either.

The authors were not formally trained and prepared to lead a department, medical school, or health science center when we started, but then most people aren't. That is the purpose of this monograph—to provide those about to enter an administrative position such as dean, department chair, center director, or division chief with some insights about the positions that will make them better administrators or at least better prepared to assume the positions and thereby to increase their longevity and effectiveness in their new roles. As most of the qualities necessary for success as an administrator are similar for all levels of leadership, we will generalize the comments to *leaders* of medical schools and single out the level of leadership (dean, chair, director, etc.) only when it is pertinent to do so.

In this book, we have provided advice in the form of "pearls of wisdom" similar to the clinical pearls we all learned in medical school. One fallacy of this approach, of course, is that no one should ever take unsolicited advice. And whether the pearls are wise may be another fallacy. Nevertheless, with a combined eighty-seven years of medical school leadership at the various levels among the three of us, we wanted to share what we have learned. We also solicited pearls from other colleagues in academic medicine and we are grateful for their contributions and have credited them when appropriate.

Chapter 1 is directed to all medical school faculty members. The pearls of this chapter deal with being a successful faculty member as well as how to preparing for being a potential medical school leader. Chapter 2 provides pearls for building a relationship with superiors and negotiating a contract. The following chapters offer pearls for adjusting to an administrative position; developing the academic missions of education, research, and clinical care; managing finances; implementing organizational change; relating to faculty and students; and dealing with the media. We then talk about things we don't like to talk about, such as how to know when we should abandon a leadership position. Finally, we apply popular management principles to academic leadership.

> We have chosen to separate the many anecdotes and quotations, for which we cannot identify a source or give credit, by a textbox so that the reader will recognize that they are not pearls.

We are indebted to our colleagues at the University of Kentucky College of Medicine and the University of Kansas School of Medicine, who taught us how to be deans and who were responsible largely for our success. And to those faculty members, students, and staff who despised us for one reason or another, we are thankful that they did not try to influence the others who were still undecided. Finally, the fact that Clara, Andrea, and Jan continue to be our wives after all these years is a tribute to their patience and tolerance, and we're grateful.

Emery A. Wilson, MD
Jay A. Perman, MD
D. Kay Clawson, MD

Contents

CHAPTER 1

Preparing to be a Medical School Leader

Young faculty members are interested primarily in teaching students, starting a research program, and, for the clinical faculty, delivering patient care. If academic medicine doesn't work out, there are always other alternatives. Basic scientists can go to industry, and clinicians can always go into private practice. Few give any thought to medical school administration. Most young faculty members are poorly prepared for becoming a faculty member much less an academic administrator.

An interest in administration is acquired as one becomes successful in academic endeavors and gains more knowledge about the university hierarchy and leadership roles and responsibilities. Some people have a natural inclination to move to leadership positions. They were class presidents or team captains in high school or college. Others become frustrated with the current leadership, and they are convinced that they would be an improvement. Still others demonstrate leadership characteristics that cause a colleague to encourage them to prepare themselves for a leadership position.

The pearls of this chapter deal with preparation for being a successful faculty member as well as a potential administrator.

> Leaders are like eagles. We don't have enough of them.

- **Learn how an academician thinks.**

The first pearl is the most difficult to explain, and that is to learn to think like an academician. Successful administrators have to appreciate the concerns of their colleagues, whether the concerns are those of education, research, or clinical service. Although it is certainly not necessary to have been a triple threat, it helps to have knowledge of each of the missions at least to the point of being able to address the issues. Having trained at or having been a faculty member at one or more major research institutions teaches one how to "think" like an academician and gives one the opportunity to develop professional relationships that can serve as valuable references when considering an administrative position.

- **Good things don't happen by accident.**

Plan, prepare, and lay the groundwork for your initiatives.

LEWIS LANDSBERG, MD
DEAN, NORTHWESTERN UNIVERSITY
FEINBERG SCHOOL OF MEDICINE

- **Take advantage of committee appointments.**

Most faculty members appointed to committees see the appointment as perfunctory or obligatory and do not do their homework. They don't read the minutes of the last meeting, they don't know the items on the agenda for the next meeting, and they are not prepared for a discussion. They resent the time away from their students and research. As in a number of other situations, in a committee meeting *knowledge is power*. If you are well prepared for the discussion during a committee meeting, you can influence the outcome of the meeting and others will think more highly of you because you are perceived to be knowledgeable about the subject matter under discussion.

> A meeting is the gathering of people who assemble to learn better how to do things they already know how to do but don't have enough time to do because they are too busy attending meetings.

- **When someone wants something, they want it now.**

We are often approached by chairs, other faculty members, or even friends asking us if we can provide information about a certain topic or if we can do something for them. Although they may say they need the information in a week or 10 days, they really want it *now*. As a courtesy, they may tell us that they want something later but they really want it now. One reason the Internet is so popular is that we can obtain information immediately instead of making a trip to the library or looking it up in a book. If you want to impress your colleagues or superiors, provide the information or complete the task requested as soon as possible, and watch the surprised look on their faces.

- **Remove the "monkey" from someone else's desk.**

Another way to impress your peers or your superiors is to take the monkey off their desk. When they come to you asking for your help, tell them that you will take care of it and they won't have to worry any longer. For example, if the dean asks you if you could possibly find the time to give a talk or arrange a conference, tell the dean that you will be happy to do so and that he/she will no longer have to worry about it, that you will take care of everything. And, again, watch the surprised look.

- **Each faculty member should be an expert in something.**

A faculty member might be an expert teacher or be knowledgeable about a rare or even a common disorder. When trying to determine an expertise, identify something that few other faculty members know about. If five thousand or even just fifty people know what you know, what you know is no longer valuable. Even if one other faculty member knows what you know, your significance in a department is less valuable. Developing a research interest and an expertise in a disease that has no known etiology or treatment distinguishes you in the field and among your peers. If your expertise is in a clinical area, an additional benefit is an increase in the number of patients requesting to see you.

> If I knew the difference between anecdote and antidote, my friend would still be alive. He was bitten by a snake and all I could do was to read him jokes from Reader's Digest. – Ron White

- **Think one level above your level in the organization.**

If you are a faculty member, try to think on the level of the chair; if you are a chair, try to think like the dean. What would your superior do in a situation like this? This helps to give you a perspective on what the person above you is thinking, and it gives your superiors and others the perception that you are a knowledgeable and mature leader.

> Bureaucracy is the process in which energy is converted into solid waste.

- **You will never be sorry for the nice things you do for people.**

There are always times when you will have to relate bad news or do things that are not popular with your peers or with those who report to you. This is inevitable, but make it a point to look for ways to "make one's day." The political capital you gain by doing nice things for others will be valuable later when you will need their understanding.

- **Make your curriculum vitae descriptive of your accomplishments.**

What do others look for in your curriculum vitae? Certainly, they look to see where you were educated, the awards you've won (especially teaching awards), your previous positions, your research funding, and your publications. Also, the types of committees you have served on can give an indication of what administrators think of you. For example, if you were selected to serve on the search committee for the medical school dean, this is evidence that you are well respected by the medical school leadership and your peers. A long list of presentations to make your curriculum vitae thicker is *not* impressive and may detract from your accomplishments.

- **Don't waste time doing research that is not likely to be published.**

If you are going to devote time to a research project, make sure that the results are important and publishable whether the results confirm or deny your hypothesis. Young faculty members often become absorbed in a project that would be spectacular if the hypothesis is confirmed but has no value if it isn't. Establishing that driving a car causes cancer would take an extraordinary effort to prove and would be a spectacular finding, but the null hypothesis is useless (for even a publication) because no one expected it to be true in the first place. On the other hand, a study of whether estrogen replacement therapy causes cancer is important if the results of the research prove the hypothesis or not.

- **When should you begin thinking about being an administrator?**

Many faculty members think they can do a better job running the department or the school than the chair or dean. Often, young faculty members who are capable or destined to be a chair think they are ready for the position before they really are. There is an element of seasoning that is necessary before taking on a leadership position. It is not necessarily age related but more related to one's ability to identify and understand the issues and problems of others and to formulate solutions. Unfortunately, succession planning is not common in academic institutions, and some find it difficult to move up within their organization. If you think you are ready, you should mention it to your superior and try to begin taking small steps toward your goal by making it known that you want to serve on a committee or become a division chief. Be mindful that other faculty members may fear your ambition and its effect on their influence if you express your desire to become an administrator, so it is sometimes better to be drafted by one's peers.

- **Do you have the characteristics of a successful administrator?**
In our previous book, *The Medical School Dean: Reflections and Directions,* we discussed the composition of a good dean. The characteristics of a successful dean or any health science administrator, in order of importance according to the contributors, were:

  1. Leadership and administrative skills
  2. Honesty, integrity, and fairness
  3. Visionary ability
  4. Ability to communicate and speak
  5. Political skills
  6. Knowledge of finances
  7. Cheerfulness and sense of humor
  8. Relationship with superiors
  9. Ability to recruit/select chairs and faculty
  10. Ability to delegate responsibility

- **Shadowing a good leader can be a valuable experience.**
Anyone interested in an administrative position should take the opportunity to shadow a dean, chair, or center director at the same or at another institution. Each day is taken up with staff, faculty, and student meetings; breakfast, lunches, and dinners; talks and presentations; community activities; and social occasions. There is little time to think and reflect. A shadowing experience can provide an important and sometimes different perspective about the position and its responsibilities.

> The key to leadership is having the capacity to know whether and when to listen to the advice of others.

- **Develop business experience.**
Because academic medical centers are becoming more corporate in nature and because school finances are diverse, many potential leaders are becoming better prepared by taking business courses in management, accounting, and finance. Some even obtain a master's degree in business administration. This is certainly not necessary to be successful, but such training may be helpful and may be seen as an asset by search committees.

- **When being considered for a medical school administrative position:**
  1. Have someone (a prominent person in the field, if possible) nominate you for the position.
  2. When contacted, write a cogent letter of application that demonstrates your knowledge of the institution and states why you believe you are qualified for the position.

3. Do your homework. Learn as much as you can about the institution, college, department, or center for which you are being considered.
4. Be prepared to state why you want the position.
5. Prepare a verbal presentation for the search committee that demonstrates your knowledge of the position and academic unit, the needs of the program, and some thoughts about what can be accomplished if you were offered the position.
6. Be prepared to give an example of how you have (or would have) handled a difficult situation.
7. Prepare some cogent questions to ask the search committee and the person responsible for the search.

- **Those who say it can't be done should shut up and get out of the way of those who are doing it.**

- **The underlying secret to success in academic administration, as in any other field of endeavor, is** *passion.*

Passion is essential for success as a student and as a faculty member, and it is essential for success as a leader.

- **It's OK to be angry at times.**

Just don't say or do something stupid while you are angry. You never know who will be on your promotions committee.

> A dean asked a faculty candidate about his strengths. The candidate said he had won 5 teaching awards, had 4 NIH grants and was in the process of discovering a cure for cancer. The dean was amazed and asked if he had any faults. "Well," said the candidate, "I have been known to exaggerate a bit."

CHAPTER 2

Negotiating a Contract

Most applicants have never negotiated for an administrative position before. In the negotiating process, keep in mind that you should first focus on building a lasting relationship with your superior, then securing the resources for the academic unit, and finally fulfilling personal needs. Many candidates for a position see negotiating as a win or lose situation. To the contrary, negotiating must be a "win-win" process, and this doesn't necessarily mean a 50-50 outcome. It is important for it to be "win-win" because you may be working with the other person for many years. This process is an opportunity for you to show your superior that you are honest, that you can justify your requests, and that you are a team player.

When searching for an administrator, the person initiating the search usually has in mind the resources necessary for the type of person to be recruited. Search committees often request this information because it is thought that it might be helpful in identifying the right candidate. On the other hand, in many cases, additional resources can almost always be identified if an applicant turns out to be the ideal candidate. So when you are in the position of being hired, don't be discouraged by what a search committee may say is the minimum or maximum recruitment package. This chapter suggests pearls for negotiating a contract when you are the candidate.

> The ability to reconcile disparate elements into a sensible solution is the hallmark of a skilled manager. To do so with grace is the gift of a true leader.

- **Identify the needs of the academic unit and develop a resource plan.**

Many people either try to negotiate for all the resources they need at the time of their appointment to a new position (because they are told that is the only way to get anything) or they don't ask for enough because they are too anxious to have the position. Identify what the current needs are and ask for those. Then inform the person with whom you are negotiating that you will later need additional resources to develop new programs to take the school or department to the next level. Consider the following approach: "These are the resources (faculty positions, space, startup funds, etc.) I need within the next year or two to bring the department/school up to national standards. Then, once I am here for a couple of years and once I have a better understanding of what is needed to take the unit to the next level, I will want to come back to you with a proposal for the resources to accomplish that. I hope you will continue to support me at that time."

> When you actually believe that you can compensate for lack of skills by doubling your efforts, there is no end to what you can't do.

- **Be knowledgeable about salary profiles.**

Use national data such as the Association of American Medical Colleges dean and faculty salary profiles to establish a salary range. Be prepared to argue for a higher salary if necessary because adjustments in university salaries are usually difficult after the initial appointment. Bonuses based on certain productivity outcomes are becoming more accepted.

- **Know the reporting structure.**

Do you report to the president, vice president, provost, dean, or chair? If you are a candidate for dean, you should have access to the president of the university. Accreditation standards for some disciplines, such as medicine, require it.

> Sometimes you may wonder why you are not receiving a superior's answer to your question or request. Often, the person responding needs to be reminded, but sometimes, it is important to understand that to not receive an answer is an answer.

- **Try to find out the real reasons the previous person has left the position.**

Sometimes the former administrator died, retired, became ill, or left for a better opportunity. However, this is not always the case, and knowing why the former administrator left might expose difficulties with superiors, lack of resources, or a recalcitrant faculty—all reasons that might cause you to be more reflective and cautious about taking the position.

- **Include the divorce arrangements at the time of the marriage.**

In addition to negotiating personal salary and other resources at the time of appointment, structure an exit plan and salary whether the exit comes in three years or thirty. Applicants are usually reluctant to talk about an exit strategy. Many in administrative positions should or would like to step down at some point but often have no place to go. Put in the contract that when you step down your salary will continue at the same amount or revert to some specified level and that you will be offered a tenured faculty position in your discipline, health policy position, etc.

- **Get a commitment that your academic unit will be a priority for the university.**

Know what the president and trustees' plans are for the school. Is your unit a priority for strategy and funding?

> A dean found a magic lamp and when he rubbed it, the emerging genie offered him his choice of infinite wealth, wisdom or beauty. Only after he chose wisdom did he realize that he should have taken the money.

CHAPTER 3

Dispelling the Myths of Academic Medicine

Like any other profession or discipline, academic medicine has adopted a number of beliefs that have become established practices over the years. Some of these practices are acknowledged to be valuable in furthering one's career and others not. The formative years in preparation for a leadership career should not be bogged down by blind acceptance of some of the mythology associated with academic medicine. The pearls of this chapter relate to the myths of academic medicine and how to avoid them in developing a career as a leader and as a faculty member.

- **Myth: The leaders of academic medicine are only those in administrative positions.**

While we often think of leadership positions in academic medicine as being confined to division chief, department chair, dean, or beyond, a much broader view of leadership is appropriate. All who aspire to be directors of a laboratory, a project, or a program will assume a leadership role. Those who serve as principal investigators on a grant are leading a team. Yet, most junior faculty members are not actively prepared and readied for leading. Faculty members should seek opportunities to participate in leadership activities beyond their specific academic focus.

- **Myth: A faculty member should avoid engaging in activities outside his/her specific interests.**

Junior faculty members are too often encouraged to make a standard policy of saying "no" when asked to serve on a committee or task force during their formative years. There is no question that growth in one's academic career requires focus on principal tasks, but it is possible to focus while finding activities to which one can say "yes." For those aspiring to be leaders, blanket "no's" result in passing up opportunities to gain knowledge of the academic medicine environment and to have valuable interactions with senior faculty and medical school leaders. Too often and particularly disappointing, junior faculty members are encouraged by mentors to limit the time they give to teaching. Saying "no" as a standard modus operandi too often portrays an image of selfishness and poor institutional citizenship and may result in the faculty member being viewed as a poor candidate for leadership in the future. Follow the advice of politician Newt Gingrich by saying "Yes, if" rather than "No, because." In other words, consider other activities in which you can become involved (teaching, committees, etc.) if certain conditions are met rather than refusing every opportunity.

- **Myth: "You should do it this way because I did it this way."**

Generational differences exist between young faculty members today and those faculty members a generation ago. Science itself requires an even greater time commitment than it did thirty years ago. And just as important, many in the current generation have legitimate differences from those in the previous generation in what they perceive to be appropriate work and personal life balances. These lifestyle requirements often leave less discretionary time for additional institutional or community service-related activities. However, if one aspires to be a leader, one should not view these additional "tasks" as purely discretionary.

- **Myth: You cannot be nice and aspire to be successful or a leader.**

"You're too nice. You're not like the rest of them." This was stated to one of us during the formative years. At the time, these words were discouraging to someone who aspired to a career in academic medicine, let alone any consideration of leadership. Why does being nice too often make a bad impression in academic medicine? The seeming weakness associated with being nice is not limited to academic medicine; the disdain for being nice pervades our culture. It is often synonymous with being a wimp: "Nice guys finish last." As physicians, the aversion to being nice creeps into our early socialization and training. We seem to lose our capacity to be nice during medical school or early in residency. Early in our careers, we become as cynical and as coarse as the rest of society. Happily, "nice" seems to be making a comeback in the business world and perhaps in academic medicine as well. Consider the recent texts: *The Power of Nice: How to Conquer the Business World with Kindness* (Thaler and Koval, 2006) and *The Power of Nice: How to Negotiate So Everyone Wins* (Shapiro and Jankowski, 1998, 2001). In *Getting to Yes*, Fisher and Ury (1981) argue that nice guys finish first. The role of the physician is to serve, not to be served.

- **Myth: You have to keep moving to different medical schools to move up the academic ladder.**

Academic medicine fails to value continuity of leadership to the degree seen in business. A conventional wisdom has emerged that new ideas and significant change are unlikely to come from insiders. Given this, it is understandable why aspiring leaders within academic medicine believe they must move from institution to institution to be promoted. Those faculty members early in their careers who want to be leaders should assess the culture of their institution regarding promoting from within. Ideally, the institution does make succession planning a priority when appropriate. If so, the notion that one needs to move from one institution to another in order to move up the ladder becomes a myth.

The value of succession planning can be found in *Built to Last* by Collins and Porras (1997), who studied the leadership of two well-known companies that had different philosophies about recruiting leaders from within their organizations. Procter & Gamble, which has had a decades-long policy of recruiting from within, grew twice as fast and had four times the profit of Colgate, which routinely recruited leaders from outside the company. Much more succession planning is needed at all administrative levels in academic medicine. Like the corporate example, those recruited from the outside are often not familiar with the organizational structure, financial processes, and culture of the school. The cost and potential deterioration in morale accompanying a prolonged national search are additional reasons for promoting from within.

That said, succession planning at some institutions means having to move. The tradition for some of the more established institutions is to hire most if not all administrators from other schools. If this is true at your institution, you must determine what position you desire at that institution and when it is most appropriate during your career for you to move to another institution and when you should apply for the position based on your credentials and your age. One way to think about this is: "As long as the institution is helping to promote my career, I will stay. When the time comes that my career is promoting the institution, I will leave." Professional accomplishments and timing are keys to obtaining an administrative position at these schools.

To err is human; to forgive is not university policy.

CHAPTER 4

Adjusting to the Position

Moving from a faculty position into administration requires a period of adjustment for you, for your former faculty colleagues, and for your new associates. You are now relating to people on an entirely different level, and that can be difficult, frustrating, and stressful. It's important to assume the role and responsibilities of the new position while retaining the personal characteristics that made you an attractive candidate and qualified for the position in the first place.

There are some things that come only with experience. Getting to the point where you feel comfortable in an administrative position takes time. Part of the comfort level relates to personal interactions, while other parts relate to developing certain management skills to be successful in the position. The following pearls can help you adjust in your new position.

> Our main business is not to see what lies dimly at a distance, but to do what lies clearly at hand. – Sir William Osler

- **The differences between leaders and managers:**
A manager administers; a leader innovates.
A manager is a copy; a leader is an original.
A manager maintains; a leader develops.
A manager focuses on structure; a leader focuses on people.
A manager relies on control; a leader inspires trust.
A manager has a short-range view; a leader has a long-range perspective.
A manager asks how and when; a leader asks what and why.
A manager has an eye on the bottom line; a leader has an eye on the horizon.
A manager imitates; a leader originates.
A manager accepts the status quo; a leader challenges it.
A manager does things right; a leader does the right thing.

- **An administrator must be a leader and a manager.**
If a leader is a person who does the right thing and a manager is a person who does things right, medical school administrators today must be both.

- **The core elements of any leader's job are academics, money, space, philanthropy and interpersonal relationships.**
A leader should be knowledgeable about the workings and dynamics of these elements, but no matter how sophisticated your skills are, hire wisely and let others manage, and do not micromanage while always demanding accountability.

Celebrate the achievements of these other managers regularly. Value philanthropy. It is the only real source of unrestricted capital. Personally create compelling institutional case statements and market them broadly to anyone who will listen. Value public presentation of the societal good that academic medicine provides. Also, communicate verbally and in writing to anyone and listen to the faculty members. They will tell you more often than not the solution to a problem no matter how complex. Most critical is to respond to them personally and with appreciation. Such personal relationships enable friendship and respect, which establishes solid institutional foundations that are apt to be durable.

PETER J. DECKERS, MD
DEAN, UNIVERSITY OF CONNECTICUT SCHOOL OF MEDICINE

> A dean or chair should be able to walk on water ... just do not disturb the fish.

- **Talk about the vision at every opportunity.**
Always be positive about the school and talk about the vision you have for the school, department, or unit. After a while, people will start to believe it.

- **Start networking immediately.**
Schedule visits to several selected schools that you believe are similar to yours (e.g., public vs. private, similar in size and scope of programs). Many organizations conduct leadership and management programs for administrators in their disciplines. For example, medical school deans should attend the Association of American Medical Colleges (AAMC) academic development seminar (deans' charm school). It is an opportunity to discuss leadership principles, meet new deans, and glean sage advice from experienced deans.

- **Identify a confidant.**
The first few months in the position can be very difficult. Everybody wants something, and every decision is good for some and unpopular with others. It is good to identify a confidant—someone to whom you can talk, curse, and yell, and know that the information will not leave the room. This can be a colleague at the school or at another school where you have already been networking. An executive coach also can be a valuable confidant.

> Leadership is the ability to hide your panic from others.

- **Be honest.**
Honesty contains power that you can use to your advantage. You certainly needn't tell everything to everybody. In fact, in many situations, the less said the better. But when you do speak, make it a habit to tell the truth. Being chronically honest has several big advantages. First, it is respectful to yourself and others. It gives people the information they need to do what they need to do, which may include helping you. Second, telling the truth is easier than lying because you don't have to remember which fabrication you told to whom.

Lies, like pigeons, have a way of coming back to you, sometimes being more trouble than they are worth. And third, people are more likely to tell you the truth when you are straight with them. As dean, I cannot always tell people what they want to hear. Sometimes I have to provide feedback that is not particularly pleasing to the recipient. In the long run, the truth is usually far more valuable for all concerned.

DONALD E. WILSON, MD, MACP
DISTINGUISHED PROFESSOR AND DEAN EMERITUS
UNIVERSITY OF MARYLAND

- **Manage your time. Beware of the "monkey" on your desk.**

There never seems to be enough time. You have to delegate responsibilities along with the authority and accountability to accomplish the task. There is a fine line between delegating and dumping. Delegating means assigning a task to a responsible person and following up periodically to make sure it is being accomplished. Dumping is making someone else do something just because you don't want to do it. Everyone will want you to take responsibility for something, and it is hard not to say that you will do something personally, but you must learn to put the "monkey" on the desk of others and not on yours. This applies to faculty and staff as well as to alumni or others from outside the institution. For example, an alumnus may call inquiring about how to get football tickets or a similar mundane topic. Your first instinct is to say that you will call the athletics department to find out the ticket policy, but you manage your time better and keep the monkey off your desk by giving the alumnus the phone number for the athletics department and letting him call for his own tickets.

- **Read as much as you can about the subject in question.**

The first year is a learning year in which you should learn about all the issues that have surfaced in the past. You will be spending a lot of weekends just reading about issues so that you can participate in the discussions and make decisions later in the week. Burn the midnight oil in the office, not at home. It is tempting to take work home but this only interferes with family life. If you must put in late hours, do so in the office so that your constituents will recognize your hard work and long hours.

- **Don't rush judgments.**

There is always time to think. If after analyzing an issue, you remain unconvinced, go with your instincts honed by a career in academia. Never forget your core values and the academic mission.

GERALD S. LEVEY, MD
DEAN, UCLA, DAVID GEFFEN SCHOOL OF MEDICINE

- **Set a timeline to make a decision.**

Everyone wants a decision … now. But most people would also be happy just knowing that they will get a decision in a timely manner. Be like an obstetrician. When a patient is in a difficult labor, a good obstetrician will set a time limit for delivery by saying, "If she doesn't progress toward delivery by a certain time, I am going to do a cesarean section." Set a time limit for a decision and then make your decision known to the person requesting it by saying, "I need to check on some things. I will give you a decision by noon on Thursday." And watch for the surprised reaction. Don't get into the habit of using the "pocket veto," that is, saying no by not answering.

- **Not making a decision is worse than making the wrong decision.**
When faced with making a decision, think of three things: *Should I? Can I? Will I?* Should I choose to go a particular direction is based on the institutional values, mission, and vision. *Can I* afford to do this with the financial and human resources available? *Will I* do this now or later (depending very often on external factors)?

PAUL ROTH, MD
DEAN, UNIVERSITY OF NEW MEXICO SCHOOL OF MEDICINE

- **Visit key administrators, chairs, and faculty members in their office.**
After your appointment, your first visits should be to others in a similar position to you. Then expand to faculty and other key administrators, particularly chairs and center directors. You can learn where their offices are and can meet faculty and staff. Meet with the administrators of departments or divisions first and identify the needs and concerns of their faculties before meeting with the entire faculty of that unit. This approach gets you out of the "ivory tower." Meet with each academic unit under your administration at least twice each year to give an update on activities and plans, and to seek their comments.

- **Feel free to call others for advice or help.**
Most chairs or deans do not like to ask for help. Yet, all counterparts are willing to provide help. When the AAMC Leadership Committee asked medical school deans if they would like to be mentored, no one responded, but almost everyone said they would be willing to be a mentor. Call them. Consultants also are particularly helpful when you need a confidant or an external resource to stimulate change. It helps when your consultants have some knowledge of your problems or have faced similar problems in other institutions.

> It's OK to be paranoid. It just means that you have a heightened awareness of your environment.

- **Surround yourself with the right people.**
When recruiting, if you haven't found the "right" person, keep looking. While academic and administrative criteria are important, personal characteristics are very important. One way to judge a recruit is to ask, "Is this someone I would enjoy having to my house for dinner?" For various reasons, an administrator is often pressured to appoint someone to a position, but appointing the right person is more important even if it takes longer.

If the wrong people are in place or if the right people are in the wrong positions, make a change as soon as you are confident that a change needs to be made. Delaying their termination is a disservice to them, to those who have to work with them, to the school, and to you.

- **Surround yourself with good people and acknowledge their successes.**

GERALD S. LEVEY, MD
DEAN, UCLA, DAVID GEFFEN SCHOOL OF MEDICINE

- **Value loyalty, but beware of blind trust.**

Part of loyalty is trust and knowing that you can depend on those around you is crucial. But a cautionary note: the blind loyalty of someone who tells you only what you want to hear is deception, and loyalty without competence is dangerous. Both will lead you down a path of ruin.

PAUL ROTH, MD
DEAN, UNIVERSITY OF NEW MEXICO SCHOOL OF MEDICINE

Never attribute to malice what can be explained by incompetence or ignorance.

- **Try to establish early in your career what your legacy will be.**

This is difficult to do at the beginning. Often your legacy is established only after you have completed your tenure in the position. However, if you can determine through good investigation and planning what is possible and what resources are available, it helps to focus your strategies to accomplish your goals. What resources do you bring? What can you offer to the institution? Consultants may help to identify your goals and what can be accomplished within the available resources.

- **Develop an appropriate format for the strategic plan.**

Strategic plans have many different formats. Consider organizing the plan into three categories: goals, objectives, and strategies. Goals are broad, overarching aspirations that relate to the mission and vision of the school. For example, a goal might be to double the research productivity within a certain timeframe. Objectives relate to the general means by which the goal will be achieved such as in this case, recruiting research-oriented faculty members. The strategies then are the specific tactics or ways by which each objective will be accomplished: solicit endowments for research chairs and professorships, involve successful research faculty in the search for new faculty members, provide a financial incentive for research faculty members who are successful in getting a new grant, etc. Identifying a person responsible for each strategy and a timeline in which it should be carried out is part of the planning process. Then there should be periodic evaluation of the plan's progress.

- Invest in the future after a well-conceived, broad-based strategic plan.

GERALD S. LEVEY, MD
DEAN, UCLA, DAVID GEFFEN SCHOOL OF MEDICINE

- **Give credit and take blame.**

Mistakes are going to happen, and no one wants to make mistakes. If the right people are in place, give them credit for everything and they will work even harder. If they make a mistake, take the blame for not giving the correct directions and they will always be loyal to you because you supported them.

- **You can always blame your predecessor, but only once.**

It's all right, even expected, to blame your predecessor when trouble arises early in your tenure. However, you must choose your issue carefully as you only get one bite of that apple. Repeated attempts to do so will backfire as they will impair your image as a strong leader.

NORMAN H. EDELMAN, MD
DEAN EMERITUS, NEW YORK STONY BROOK UNIVERSITY
SCHOOL OF MEDICINE

> The secret to success is knowing who to blame for your failures.

- **Smile a lot.**

Faculty and staff like to think things are going well. No one likes bad news. You will spend a lot of your time describing reality, which may not be good, but everyone wants to hear about the solution, not the problem. The mood of the faculty is often a reflection of your mood. If you maintain a pleasant demeanor, it helps create a sense of well-being.

- **To the extent possible, do not conduct business in your office.**

Always go to see the person that you want to speak with in his/her office, laboratory, or clinic. When you invite someone to your office, you are sending the nonverbal message that you are very important and that the person needs to disrupt his day and routine to come see you. When, in contrast, you go to see a person on his own turf, you are sending the message that he is important and that what he has to say is so crucial to you that you have disrupted your routine to seek him out. This may give you an advantage in any negotiations that ensue. It is, in addition, worthwhile to conduct your business outside of your office so that you can get a feel of the physical facilities in which your faculty, colleagues, and students are working.

EDWARD C. HALPERIN, MD
DEAN, UNIVERSITY OF LOUISVILLE SCHOOL OF MEDICINE

- **Don't allow faculty members to go over your head without your knowledge.**

Faculty members and chairs often like to talk directly to the president or vice president about things that concern them. You should support academic freedom, but it is also a courtesy to you that you know when someone is talking to those above you in the university hierarchy and what they are talking about. At least then you will know about the problem when the president asks you about it. This often needs to be enforced when you first take office (because a former dean, vice president, or president allowed it) and reinforced any time you find it occurring.

- **Have a sense of humor but beware of jokes.**

Nothing defuses a difficult situation like a sense of humor. Knowing when to use humor and when not to is a challenge. It helps to use self-deprecating humor when at all possible. On the other hand, many jokes offend someone. If you ever wonder or ask yourself whether or not you should tell a joke because it might be offensive, don't tell it. In other words, when in doubt, don't.

- **Everything you say will be taken seriously ... by someone.**
People hear what they want to hear, and it often differs from person to person or in context. It always seems that when you are being serious, someone will think it's a joke. And when you are trying to be humorous, you can always count on someone to take it seriously.

- **Don't talk about chairs or faculty members to others.**
Chairs or faculty members rightly assume that if you are talking *to* them about others, you are also talking *about* them to others. And don't think that chairs or faculty members don't talk to each other about what you said or about what resources you have committed to them.

- **Always do what you say you will do or provide a reason why.**
Over time, other administrators and the faculty appreciate a leader who is honest, trustworthy, and especially one who will carry through on commitments. They also know that it is not always possible to do everything one promises, but when it doesn't happen, they deserve to know why. Occasionally, someone *thinks* you promised something when you didn't. If at all possible, fulfill the promise they believe you made to them. If they really believe that you made the promise and they feel that strongly about it, it is better to retain your credibility and their support than to be right.

- **When you are discouraged, reflect on why you were hired in the first place.**
Administrators can often have a personality change after being in the office a while. We think we are too important or too powerful. When things aren't going right, we don't understand why people don't agree with us or like us. That's the time to get away, walk on the beach, or go for a hike. Try to restore your true personality. That's why you were hired.

- **Accept every invitation the first year. Then, you can be more selective.**
The first year in an administrative position is difficult. Everyone wants your time. They want you to attend seminars, department meetings, faculty meetings, dinner parties, and holiday events. Try to attend as many meetings and events as possible during the first year. After the first year, you might delegate some meetings to associates, or go to only certain parties, or go alternate years, etc. During the holidays, you soon learn to show up at a party, mingle among the crowd for ten or fifteen minutes (to be seen), and then go to the next party.

- **Recognize your strengths and weaknesses, and delegate your weaknesses.**
No one is good at everything. Learn what you are good at and delegate your weaknesses to an associate. Negotiating with a chair or faculty candidate is a good example. Candidates often ask for more resources than the school can possibly provide because that is what they have been taught, and yet they may be attracted for far less. Some administrators may be good at negotiating start-up packages and others not. If you are not, find an associate who is good at negotiating, provide the guidelines for the negotiation, and let him or her negotiate with the candidate. Delegation can be a form of mentoring and succession planning. Delegation of responsibilities applies also to office

staff, such as sorting the mail, screening electronic mail, and drafting letters for signature.

> Tenacity is a virtue; stubbornness is a vice. Know when to cut your losses.

• **When you are overwhelmed, make a list.**
When you find yourself in a situation where you have multiple tasks to do and you hardly know where to start, make a list of the tasks and check off each one when it is completed. This gives you a sense of accomplishment and progress toward their completion.

> If it weren't for stress, I would have no energy at all.

• **You are seldom complimented for what you do.**
Your reward is seeing others excel.

> Successful leaders are those who learn to manage disappointment.

• **It's hard not to agree with the following four management principles:**
Choose very good people.
Delegate appropriate authority to them.
Know the facts and admit what you don't know.
Be honest.

• **As a leader, continue to do what you do best.**
If you have been an educator, continue to teach; pursue research if you are a scientist; deliver patient care if you are a clinician. Be disciplined. Carve out dedicated time weekly to establish presence in one of these domains. Be continuously engaged and committed and be public about it; it will root your total activity as a leader in real institutional and community credibility that will win the respect of all faculty and staff. Such effort may also be good for your mental health.

PETER J. DECKERS, MD
DEAN, UNIVERSITY OF CONNECTICUT SCHOOL OF MEDICINE

• **Don't deplete yourself.**
Depletion yields depression or erratic behavior.

• **A dean's job is to solve problems.**
At the end of the day, the dean's job is to solve the problems that keep chairs and faculty members from succeeding. Of course, one person's solution is another's problem. This is not easy to explain. When my children ask what I do, I answer, "I solve problems. Every day I try to solve more problems than I create, and I don't always have good days."

THOMAS A. DEUTSCHE, MD
DEAN, RUSH MEDICAL COLLEGE

- **Multidisciplinary centers are difficult to manage.**

A center director probably has the most difficult administrative position because a center is essentially a matrix organization. It is not a part of the typical college/department organizational structure but, by definition, has faculty members from several departments working on a particular problem. Not only do the faculty members report to someone else (their respective chairs), but the center director often may have to report to more than one superior (e.g., dean, vice president, provost). Since this is a schizophrenogenic reporting structure, a center director must be relatively mature and comfortable with ambiguity.

- **Time and appointment management are necessary to carry out the expectations and responsibilities of the position.**

A diplomatic executive assistant who can triage faculty, students, visitors, and mail can be a valuable asset. Because of demands on time, an administrator should program certain activities such as meeting with students and faculty into the daily or weekly agenda in order to prevent being isolated from one's constituents.

- **Time away from the institution can restore perspective.**

Leadership positions can be emotionally and physically draining. Sometimes the stress of constant confrontation and the fiduciary responsibility can even cause personality changes. Time away to visit other institutions or attend meetings with colleagues is valuable, but vacation time is most important to restore perspective.

- **Complacency is the handmaiden of mediocrity.**

Even strong programs can always be better. A dispassionate look is a prerequisite for success.

LEWIS LANDSBERG, MD
DEAN, NORTHWESTERN UNIVERSITY
FEINBERG SCHOOL OF MEDICINE

- **Don't ever think people are creating problems for you in this job.**

The job is problems, and your job is to solve them (or tell them they are insoluble and move on).

RICHARD D. KRUGMAN, MD
DEAN, UNIVERSITY OF COLORADO SCHOOL OF MEDICINE

Leader's Lament
  I'm not allowed to run the train
  Or see how fast it will go.
  I'm not allowed to let off steam
  And make the whistle blow.
  I cannot exercise control
  Or even ring the bell,
  But let the damn thing jump the track
  And see who catches hell!

CHAPTER 5

Realizing that Education is the Priority

Caring for others is what attracted most of us to the field of medicine, but teaching the next generation of health professionals will be our enduring legacy. There is no finer task. Treating a patient with a rare disorder brings immediate satisfaction, but teaching a skill or imparting special knowledge can have an effect on generations of health professionals and their patients. Although the presence of students may slow our care of patients, most health professionals consider teaching an obligation and a pleasure. Teaching is also an important learning process for the teacher.

Education in the clinical disciplines has changed significantly during the past century. What was once an apprenticeship model of teaching evolved to more of a full-time faculty model in many schools, although the community-based faculty still provides a large amount of clinical education. Now, regulatory activities (the Health Insurance Portability and Accountability Act [HIPAA], coding, etc.) have increased the administrative burden for health professionals, resulting in more frustration and decreased time spent with students. For the clinical faculty, increased productivity expectations have further compromised their contributions to the other academic missions. Nevertheless, what sustains the great physician now and in the future is the opportunity to teach young doctors how to care for others.

The following pearls identify ways to promote the education mission and to reward our best teachers.

> Medical education must be built around caring to learn and learning to care.

- **Focus on curriculum design, innovation, oversight, and evaluation.**
There are experts in all aspects of education, and it would be helpful if you had at least one in curriculum development and assessment and one in student/resident evaluation. Beware of the academic staff you inherit. They may not be current in what directions the curriculum needs to go.

- **In the education mission, focus on process as well as outcome.**
Some educators are content to accept graduation rates or results on board/licensure examinations as determinants of success of an educational program. But as W. Edward Deming demonstrated in Japan's postwar reconstruction, if you want to improve the outcome, improve the process. For this reason, accreditation agencies are now focusing on process as much as or more than outcome. The same management concept may be applied to the clinical or research missions.

- **Maintain ongoing compliance with accreditation standards.**

One of the worst things for a school (and for the dean) or for a department (and for the chair) is to lose accreditation. Accreditation tends to be the last thing an administrator thinks about until it is time for an accreditation site visit. Read and understand the accreditation standards and select someone to maintain compliance with the standards. Periodically review all the accreditation standards, whether or not the school or department is in compliance with the standard, and the evidence for compliance. The faculty and staff will often say that the school or program is in compliance with a standard when it is not, so demand the evidence for compliance. Consider having an internal or external consultant review your compliance with the standards midway through the accreditation cycle.

- **Education is the least expensive way to develop national prominence.**

Several schools or departments have established a national reputation based on their curriculum and pedagogy. It is much less expensive and time-consuming to develop a national reputation in education than building a reputation in the research or clinical enterprises.

> I think this is the most extraordinary collection of talent, of human knowledge, that has ever been gathered at the White House with the possible exception of when Thomas Jefferson dined alone. – John F. Kennedy at a White House dinner for Nobel laureates

- **Teaching students is the only thing that a medical school does that is not performed by some other entity.**

Teaching hospitals can have residency training programs, research institutes can do research, and private practitioners can provide care, but only medical schools have the responsibility of educating medical students and granting MD degrees. The dean and in part all leaders need to reinforce this to the faculty, who understandably tend to focus more on research or patient care. The dean must be the advocate for the education of students, and a good chair or division chief understands the need to promote the educational mission of the school. Everything we do in clinical care and research should create a better educational environment for our students.

- **Promote active learning.**

Many accreditation committees are interested in both the process of education as well as the outcome, and they are encouraging more active learning by students rather than passively listening to lectures and feverishly taking notes. Because of the amount of information available, students should be taught how to learn and retrieve the information they need. The pedagogy that best imparts the information being taught—lectures, small group teaching, case-based learning, problem-based learning, computer-based learning, simulated patients, or other pedagogy—is the one that should be used, and a variety of pedagogies should be encouraged.

> When asked whether his problems were due to ignorance or apathy, one student said, "I don't know and I don't care."

- **Each academic unit should identify or recruit a master teacher.**

If a department has one teacher who is considered to be outstanding by the students, the whole department often is perceived to be good in education. Students value most the time that is spent with them. For that reason, each department should have at least one excellent teacher. Chairs should consider recruiting a faculty member for teaching skills in the same way they recruit for research or clinical skills.

> Trying to teach a pig is not only difficult but it is very frustrating for the pig.

- **Listen to the students.**

Use periodic meetings with students, student evaluation of courses and instructors, and surveys or questionnaires to find out what's really going on in the curriculum.

- **You cannot compliment or reward great teachers enough.**

Look for ways to promote teaching and teachers. Some schools have developed "academies" or "centers" of education that bring together educators of different disciplines in order to stay abreast of curricular changes and newer pedagogies and to establish a common bond among the teaching faculty similar to multi-disciplinary research centers. Great teaching can also be rewarded through the promotion and tenure process, salary adjustments, awards, and public recognition.

- **Consider mission-based management/budgeting as a means to empha-size teaching.**

Mission-based management and budgeting is a method used to assign faculty effort to one of the three missions and then fund each faculty position based on the amount of time spent teaching, doing research, or caring for patients. This method has been used effectively to identify and target institutional funds for rewarding the teaching effort of the faculty as well as for other mission efforts. At a minimum, emphasize that a portion of faculty compensation is in fact tied to the education mission.

> During the past month, I have had an LCME site visit and I have had a colonoscopy. I'll leave it to you to decide which prep was the most difficult.
>
> RONALD D. FRANKS, MD
> VICE PRESIDENT FOR HEALTH SCIENCES
> UNIVERSITY OF SOUTH ALABAMA

CHAPTER 6

Developing and Growing Research

For universities, there are only a few big pools of money that provide revenue streams, and one of them is medical research funding from the National Institutes of Health, National Science Foundation, pharmaceutical companies, and related foundations. These research sources provide more than $80 billion annually, and a major portion of that funding is allocated to universities. Therefore, universities and health science schools in particular should position themselves to pursue these sources of funding.

Many schools have a history of research productivity while others need essentially to start from the beginning. Remember that research can be performed in education as well as in the basic and clinical sciences. The pearls in this chapter focus on developing research strengths and the best use of research resources.

- **Focus on research strengths and invest in them.**

No school or department can excel in everything no matter how large the program may be. Identify the program's strengths in one or more missions and build around them. Unfortunately, every school is trying to build strengths in hot-button areas such as cardiovascular sciences, neurosciences, and cancer. We all have a tendency to develop a strength and then ignore it while trying to build strengths in another areas. Remember that no academic unit ever stays at the same level. It is always either improving or diminishing, so administrators must continue to invest in an area in order for it to continue to be a strength.

> Ignoring the facts does not change the facts.

- **Learn from industry.**

Universities and academic units can improve their operations by employing some of the principles used in successful corporations. Jim Collins's (2001) book, *Good to Great,* distinguishes the characteristics of several "great" companies from others that he classifies as good but not great. He focuses on leadership development, selecting the right people, confronting the brutal facts that need to be addressed, focusing on a few things that a company does better than any other, and developing a culture of discipline that not only allows the company's personnel to excel but also prevents distractions from interfering with what the company does best. Academic institutions could benefit from adopting similar characteristics.

> At a meeting of the Harvard overseers, they were asked to review the university's 26 worthy goals. The then chair of Monsanto said, "I'm only a soap salesman, but if you want to accomplish anything worthwhile, select 3 or 4 goals and achieve them."

- **Build research in the basic sciences first if you are starting from the beginning.**

Once you have strength in one or more of the basic sciences, it is easier to recruit clinicians to work in the same area. Usually, at least three people are necessary to create a working research group, and having a core of basic scientists helps establish a stronger discipline. The distinction between basic and clinical departments is becoming less and less obvious because clinical departments are recruiting basic scientists to do research. This further supports the need to recruit basic scientists first.

- **When you have good researchers, it's easier to recruit good researchers.**

Go after a few top-notch investigators. Through their reputations and national influence, they will attract people to work with them.

- **Establish a plan for building a research program.**

You can build research by hiring young people and developing them or by hiring an established, well-funded person. The former is less expensive. An instantaneous solution in starting a research program is to hire a well-funded investigator and his/her team. However, it is very expensive and time-consuming to recruit a team that may not come if one or two members of the team eventually decide against it. As an alternative, identify a promising young person and build around him/her. Or, grow your own researchers by providing appropriate mentoring and training.

- **Look for ways for researchers to collaborate.**

Proximity breeds attempt. Putting researchers in adjacent space helps collaboration. Multidisciplinary centers encourage collaboration, increase visibility, and often enhance extramural funding. The best way to build collaboration is to appoint the right person to lead the particular research enterprise—someone who has the right personal skills and who values interdisciplinary or multidisciplinary efforts.

> To steal ideas from one person is plagiarism. To steal from many people is research. – Steven Wright

- **Make the best use of research space.**

Schools and departments take ownership of research space in the established health science center, and reallocating space from nonproductive to more productive researchers can be a challenge. Establish a policy for the use of research space based on productivity (e.g., $300 research funding per net square foot of research space, number of graduate students, etc.). It is often helpful to have a committee of highly respected and productive researchers review the space utilization and productivity in order to justify reallocation.

- **Create core facilities to maximize utilization of research methods.**

Many research techniques (e.g., cell sorting, flow cytometry, transgenic mice, etc.) may be used by multiple researchers but are too expensive for independent researchers. Establishing core facilities on a cost basis justifies these investments.

- **Create incentives for research productivity.**

Most institutions provide protected time and full faculty salaries for a period of time (e.g., three years) and then expect the faculty member to generate a portion of his/her salary from grants. Others provide financial incentives from salary reimbursements of grants. Financial awards and public recognition can also be used to reward productive researchers.

> It's a wonderful feeling when you discover some evidence to support your beliefs.

- **Develop a lucrative policy for intellectual property.**

The university rightfully can expect to benefit from the financial proceeds of intellectual property when the product is produced with university time and resources, but proceeds to the research developer of such property should be substantial in order to provide appropriate incentive.

> We have rats that die of too much of something and we have rats that die of too little of something. What we need are healthier rats. – Lou Holtz, former football coach

CHAPTER 7

Caring for Others

The mission that differs most among the nation's medical schools, as well as between the medical school and the other academic units of a university, is the clinical service mission. Accreditation standards and national standardized examinations, such as the United States Medical Licensing Examination (USMLE), have created similar educational curricula for all schools. Basic and clinical science research is similar for most schools, although there is a wide range in the magnitude of research and funding. On the other hand, the clinical enterprises of medical schools vary tremendously in size and format. Some schools are a part of a university-owned academic health center, while others depend on community hospital or veterans hospital affiliations for the education of students and care of patients. Furthermore, clinical faculty appointments range from full-time to part-time to voluntary, and all of them are valuable to the growing education and clinical research missions.

The clinical mission is also the one that has changed the most in recent history. Government reimbursement for the care of the elderly and poor through Medicare and Medicaid, corporate medicine, managed care, medical technology, and federal regulations have all had a significant impact on academic medicine. In the future, medical schools will be involved more with electronic sharing of medical information, quality of care initiatives, clinical guidelines and decreases in variation of care, and even more technological advances. Since the clinical faculty salaries depend more and more on clinical revenues, emphasis on measures of clinical productivity are likely to impinge on the capacity for faculty members to be involved in teaching and research.

The pearls in this chapter relate to caring for patients and managing the clinical enterprise.

- **Focus on clinical strengths but keep educational needs in mind.**
The same three areas that schools tend to focus on in research—cardiovascular sciences, neurosciences, and cancer—are true also for clinical care, but clinical strengths can be in any discipline as long as they generate clinical revenue. In determining which clinical programs to support or expand, consider the ones that generate the most income for the time and money invested. When enlarging or downsizing programs, remember that the school needs the core clinical activities for student education.

- **What can you do that others in private practice cannot?**
Private physicians may provide care that is just as good as that of academic physicians, and the care is usually more convenient for patients. Find disciplines,

techniques, or procedures that distinguish the academic from the private physicians in your geographic area.

> If a pretty poster or a cute saying is all that it takes to motivate you, you probably have a very easy job…one that a robot will be doing soon.

• Take a strong role in the management of clinical affairs.
If your school has full-time clinicians, you or an administrative associate should maintain a strong role in managing the clinical enterprise. This may be in conjunction with a vice president for health affairs and with a hospital director. The faculty needs to see that you have a significant clinical role. You may be head of the practice plan or group practice or you may be instrumental in directing the clinical activities through an associate dean or chair for clinical affairs, chief of staff, or clinic director. Focus on quality of care, decreasing variability of care, clinical guidelines, patient amenities, and working as a group practice.

> The dean is the shepherd of the faculty and the chairs are the crooks on which he/she leans.

• Find ways to work with hospital administration.
From a dean's or chair's perspective, the hospital is there to support the academic missions of the school. The clinical faculty and hospital administration are often at odds. Hospital administrators must be interested in the bottom line even though they want to support the academic missions. Try to work with the hospital administration to establish "win-win" outcomes. When you think about it, the university also is interested in the bottom line of the hospital, and if the hospital is doing well financially, the hospital administrator is secure in the position. Any arguments you have with hospital administration will fall on deaf ears and you will be seen as the troublemaker. So, try to work with hospital administrators. Several academic medical centers have moved to a single enterprise system that minimizes these tensions.

> Access to health care is a right. Smoking and carrying an AK47 are privileges.

• Some clinical relationships are like a marriage.

Of all the relationships a school of medicine has, the one that is most like a marriage is the one with the Veterans Administration. This is a sixty-year-old bond that has had its ups and downs, but the best way to make it work is to realize that both have much to gain by the union and that to sustain it requires mutual respect, understanding, and compromise. One cannot dominate the other, and it is a daily opportunity to find ways to complement and support the other, recognizing always that each brings a great deal to the relationship and that much would be lost if the relationship is not nurtured and improved with each passing year.

JOSEPH G. REVES, MD
DEAN, MEDICAL UNIVERSITY OF SOUTH CAROLINA
SCHOOL OF MEDICINE

- **Determine which clinical departments will be more academic and which will be primarily educational and clinical.**

Some clinical departments have weak or little interest in academic endeavors, especially research. This may be because the discipline has never developed major funding sources nationally or it may be because the faculty members in the department simply are not interested. Trying to have all departments become National Institutes of Health (NIH) powerhouses is not realistic. Some departments should have only a service and education role.

- **Identify the clinical needs of the community.**

When selecting areas of strength for investing resources, keep in mind the clinical needs of the community, especially if you are in a public school. "Diagnose" the community (state, city, etc.) ills and try to address them. It helps to build political favor.

> Good health is merely the slowest possible rate at which one can die.

- **Emphasize that the medical school needs to care for its own.**

The medical school faculty should be encouraged to care for family members, friends, and family members of the university faculty. The university faculty and staff can be among your biggest supporters.

> Some of these days, when we all die of nothing, we are going to feel pretty stupid. – Redd Foxx

- **Promote transparency among medical school, department, practice plan, and hospital stakeholders.**

Sharing of information in a transparent manner leads to trust among senior administrators. It is also important for planning and the best use of resources. Centralization of financial decision making to a committee of institutional leaders is more likely to direct resources where they are most needed, whether it be teaching simulators, additional faculty members, or a piece of hospital equipment.

> A man took his car into a garage for repairs and was told that the parts would take a while to order. "How long?" the man asked. "I can give you an appointment five years from Tuesday," said the mechanic. "In the morning or the afternoon?" asked the man. "What difference does it make?" asked the mechanic, "it's five years from now." The man replied, "I have a doctor's appointment in the afternoon."

CHAPTER 8

Keeping an Eye on the Money

If you have held an administrative position before, the budget and the budget planning process may be something with which you are familiar, but if you have not been directly involved with the budget process, it can be intimidating. Since most academic administrators have fiduciary responsibility for their academic units, careful financial management is one of their most important roles. This responsibility entails the acquisition of funds from various sources, planning the best use of funds, creating a budget, and then managing the academic unit within that budget. It is not unlike your personal bank account except there are many more sources of revenue (tuition, state or local funds, grants and contracts, practice plans, hospitals, gifts and endowments, etc.) and expense categories (personnel, equipment, space rental or construction, operating expenses, travel, utilities, etc.). Institutions are similar in the type of accounting and budgeting process they use, but they may differ in detail and method. Public institutions tend to have more restrictions and regulations on institutional funds and how they are spent. Persistent mismanagement of budgeted resources will not be tolerated by senior academic administrators and, if you are responsible for their mismanagement, neither will you. This chapter offers a few pearls about the financial aspects of an academic unit.

- **Have a budget/finance officer whom you trust implicitly.**
The person in this position should be involved in the decision making and planning of programs, but it should never be perceived that the bottom line is driving school or departmental policy. Periodic audits of financial accounts are a must for the protection of both the academic unit and the administrator. For the same reasons, financial accounts should be audited whenever there is a change in administrators.

> Fundamentally, there are only two ways of coordinating the economic activities of millions. One is central direction involving the use of coercion—the technique of the army and of the modern totalitarian state. The other is voluntary cooperation of the individuals—the technique of the marketplace. – Milton Friedman

- **The budget process is a negotiating process.**
The annual budget process in a university is more than a financial exercise. Many people call it a planning process because you are planning how you will invest your resources, and after all, if you don't put resources behind a strategy, it is unlikely to have much meaning or success. Even more significant is the

understanding that the budget is a negotiating process. The university and its constituent colleges have only so many resources, and you are competing with all the other academic units for those resources, so you are really negotiating for funds for your program. Sometimes you can be successful in getting funds by listening to what the president or other administrative superior has been emphasizing the past year. For example, if the president has been saying that the university should be more involved in international activities, become involved and "negotiate" for the resources to promote that activity.

• **Take advantage of budget reductions.**
In every crisis, there is an opportunity. Budget reductions are painful, but they also present an opportunity to eliminate some programs/departments/staff that are no longer part of the strategic plan (see Chapter 9).

• **State funds are like an endowment but…**
For public schools, state funds are important. In fact, they are like an endowment supported by the state. One million dollars in state funds is like having a $20 million endowment for private schools. On the other hand, cyclic funding reductions that follow declines in state revenues can be difficult to manage. Budget reductions of less than 5 percent can usually be taken "across the board" but to accommodate larger cuts, programmatic reductions should be considered (see Chapter 9).

• **You must know where to get money.**
An important part of any senior administrator's responsibility is not only having money but knowing how and where to get it. There are several sources for funds: tuition, state, dean's tax, clinical revenues, indirect cost dollars, salary reimbursement from grants, gifts, endowment, hospital, foundations, etc. Of equal importance is the need to build a relationship with the managers of these fund sources (e.g., the administrator of indirect cost dollars) in order to be able to acquire funding when you need it. A past history of productive use of such funding always helps.

> Henry Ford, on a visit to Ireland, agreed to give $5,000 to a hospital there. To his dismay, the hospital announced that he agreed to give $50,000. He told the hospital administrator that he would indeed give $50,000 but only if the hospital would place the following saying on a plaque: "I came unto you as a stranger, and you took me in."

CHAPTER 9

Managing a Financial Crisis

Most of us in the academic world have equated success with growth—more funding for research, more graduate students, more patients, and above all more money. We excuse our failures as lack of support from the university or the government, which usually equates to money. Uncontrolled growth, however, can spell disaster in some situations, whether in the cells of cancer or in a vineyard where selected pruning is essential for product quality.

One of us remembers well a lesson learned in Seattle during the Boeing Company crisis of the late 1960s when signs began appearing on the highways: "Will the last person to leave please turn out the lights." Two days after the Boeing layoffs were announced, another large downtown company announced major layoffs. The president of the company was asked why the Boeing situation would affect his operation so soon and he said, "It won't, but I have been waiting a long time to be able to get rid of deadwood. Now I can act without the criticism that comes with letting long-time employees go." Both companies prospered by "managing the crisis" and are larger and more successful than ever. The pearls in this chapter demonstrate how.

- **Take advantage of budget cuts or restraints to reexamine what you are doing and how you are doing it.**
When a budget cut is announced, the first tendency is to blame the source and then to begin thinking about how the reduction will be managed. There is a propensity to reduce every unit or person by the same percentage to account for the reduction. Usually, an across-the-board decrease can be accomplished if the reduction is less than 5 percent. If the budget cut is greater than this amount, a selective decrease in programs should be considered. Successive budget cuts of 5 percent or less, however, justify more significant programmatic changes. Programmatic cuts usually require the approval of superiors with a comprehensive plan for how the program reductions will be implemented. Although there is a tendency to use budget cuts to remove troublesome employees, downsizing should be focused on programs and not individuals, even though the reasons for downsizing may be, in part, individuals.

> In every crisis is an opportunity.

- **Involve employees appropriately at all levels of the organization.**
Maintaining morale during a financial downturn is difficult. When employees don't know what is happening, rumors abound. During difficult times, one cannot communicate enough. Communications can take many forms: electronic or written mail, faculty and staff conferences, and one to one.

- **Determine what can be eliminated that might result in actually improving the organization.**

First, determine those strengths of the organization that distinguish the school and should be preserved. As Jim Collins (2001) indicated in *Good to Great,* identify the school's *hedgehog concept* (major strength) and use budget reductions to promote it by eliminating programs that would otherwise interfere with it.

- **Reallocating revenues can improve productivity.**

Restructuring the school or department may actually result in increased productivity of some faculty members or staff which, in turn, may result in increased compensation for deserving personnel.

- **Maintain a positive attitude during the downsizing process.**

Crisis management requires the leader to remain positive and upbeat about what is being accomplished rather than dwelling on the cause of the crisis, who is to blame, or sympathizing with naysayers. The crisis should not be used as an excuse for past or future failure.

- **How you manage in times of budget cuts or other crises is the sign of a gifted administrator.**

As John Hogness, former president of the University of Washington and president of the Association of Academic Health Centers, often said, "It doesn't take much ability to be successful in times of increased funding. The mark of an outstanding administrator is what is accomplished in times of decreased funding."

- **Long before you have to face a crisis, build political capital.**

The leaders of the university and community (your friends) may be more important in diffusing the crisis and in your keeping your job than any other single factor. Use the time between crises to build the political capital necessary to sustain you through the bad times, financial or otherwise.

> Under certain circumstances, profanity provides a relief denied even in prayer.
> – Mark Twain

CHAPTER 10

Managing Organizational Change

Change in itself is constant in a medical school setting. We are constantly changing diagnoses and treatments. Even changing leaders—deans, chairs, directors, etc.—is usually well tolerated in a medical school. However, organizational change such as major revisions in the curriculum or practice plan creates predictable and considerable upheaval for the faculty and sometimes for students. As Machiavelli pointed out, change creates anxiety for both those who are comfortable with the old system because they may lose prestige and power and for those in the new system because their future is unpredictable.

Organizational change requires careful preparation, strong commitment of leadership, internal and external stimuli, champions of the need for change, constant communication with faculty and students, and institutionalization of the change. The following are pearls that relate to organizational change and how to implement it.

> It should be borne in mind that there is nothing more difficult to handle, more doubtful of success, and more dangerous to carry through than initiating changes…The innovator makes enemies of all those who prospered under the old order and only lukewarm support is forthcoming from those who would prosper under the new. – Niccolo Machiavelli

- **Change is the only way to improve.**
Think of change as a campaign, a planned process that requires forethought, strategy, and careful implementation.

> If you never try anything new, you will miss out on many of life's greatest disappointments.

- **Keep an eye out for best practices.**
At national meetings, look for best practices and opportunities to change or improve. Try to bring back at least one new idea from each meeting that can be implemented at your school.

> A mistake is proof that someone at least tried to accomplish something.

- **Change is difficult for everyone.**

The most difficult things to change seem to be the curriculum or a practice plan. Change can be facilitated by external pressure or by internal advocates. It often helps to have both. No matter what you want to change, 20 percent of the faculty will like it, 20 percent will hate it, and the others really won't care. Try to keep the negative faction in the 20 percent range, and you can accomplish any change you wish. But when 40 percent or more of the faculty oppose a change, reconsider.

> Meetings bore me because I already know the decision. – Joseph Stalin

- **Don't ask the faculty to endorse too much change at once.**

There is a tendency to want to make many changes all at once. Like any individual, the faculty can absorb and process only so much change within a certain timeframe. The leader of change must be able to sense when to promulgate more change versus giving the faculty a chance to take a breath.

> We should change when we see the light, not when we feel the heat.

- **Changing the curriculum is like…**

We have all heard that changing the curriculum is like moving a graveyard, but only those who have tried to make significant changes in the curriculum really know what that means. First, in order to move a graveyard, you have to know where the skeletons are, and there can be a lot of skeletons among the faculty. Once you know where the skeletons are located, you can move them very carefully so as not to disarticulate the skeletons, but sometimes you have to move them with a bulldozer … and the dean has to drive the bulldozer.

- **All great change is incremental.**

This adage was reinforced when the Clinton administration tried to change the health care system. It is difficult and often impossible to completely change large systems that are entrenched. On the other hand, purposeful and significant change can be incrementally implemented.

> Sometimes, as a leader in a medical school, you find that you need to talk to God. If you talk to God, it is called praying. If God talks to you, it is called schizophrenia.
>
> Any time I talk about change, one of our faculty members always reminds me that, in nature, most mutations are lethal.
>
> I am all for innovation; it is change that I don't like.
>
> We tend to meet any new situation by reorganizing, and what a wonderful method it can be for creating the illusion of progress while producing inefficiency and demoralization. – Petronius

CHAPTER 11

Relating to Faculty and Students

Interacting with the faculty and students is usually one of the pleasant responsibilities of a medical school leader, but there are times when it can be challenging. Leaders selected from within the organization may find it difficult to relate to the faculty, especially those in their department. Leaders often bend over backward not to favor their former department or division, often to the detriment of the faculty. Being a leader also can be a lonely job because a lot of information cannot be shared and former friends no longer relate to the new role of the leader in the same manner. Leaders selected from other institutions must identify with the culture of the new school as well as get to know the faculty, staff, and students while simultaneously learning the history of various school initiatives, planning future programs, and adjusting to the position. The pearls in this chapter focus on how to relate to faculty and students.

- **Look for ways to relate to the faculty.**

You can never communicate enough. Look for multiple ways to communicate with the faculty: faculty meetings, department meetings, Internet, dean's letters, etc. Remember, communication is a two-way process. Don't think you are effectively communicating by writing reports and sending e-mails without also providing an opportunity for feedback.

- **Treat everyone with respect.**

Keep your promises and never lose your cool. Always make yourself available for students.

GERALD S. LEVEY, MD
DEAN, UCLA, DAVID GEFFEN SCHOOL OF MEDICINE

> A professional is an ordinary person called upon to do extraordinary things. Professionalism is a character trait. – Edmund D. Pellegrino, MD

- **Administrative style is important.**

The dean needs to be able to exhibit the steely confidence of Chilli Palmer in *Get Shorty*, the decisive problem solving of Winston Wolf in *Pulp Fiction*, and the quiet and magical sincerity of Aldus Dumbledore in the *Harry Potter* series.

THOMAS A. DEUTSCH, MD
DEAN, RUSH MEDICAL COLLEGE

- **Don't expect the faculty to organize behind you.**

The faculty is disorganized by definition. Academic freedom and faculty independence ensures disorganization. That is why universities have so many regulations and such complicated hierarchies. The faculty expects you as their leader to accomplish what they need. If you approach the faculty to rise up for or against something, they will say, "That's your job." And they are probably right. Their perception, though not always verbalized, is that you are ineffective at doing your job if you have to ask them to organize around an issue.

> Consensus is what everyone believes collectively, but no one wants to say individually. – Abba Eban

- **Sometimes the faculty is right.**

If a significant percentage of the faculty is opposed to something, rethink it. The faculty may be right. If so, don't be afraid to say you were wrong. In fact, always be quick to say you are wrong when you are. Most people, including superiors, will be willing to forgive and forget, saying something like, "Oh, it wasn't your fault."

- **Don't ask a question you don't want to know the answer to.**

There are some things you really don't want to know. Medical school faculty members are entrepreneurs. As long as someone is not doing something illegal or directly disobeying a university official or regulation, you may not want to know the details of their operation. There are times when the leader might say, "I don't think I want to know about that." Similarly, there may be times when it is better for faculty or students to ask for forgiveness than for permission.

- **Dealing with difficult people should be a "snap" for a dean who is keenly interested in human behavior.**

"Snap," as it turns out, is a double entendre. The first meaning is the innocent meaning, that is, as a psychiatrist I should have certain skill sets that enable me to work with just about anyone, including faculty members and administrators. The satiric meaning refers to the sharp "snap" of the neck when confronted by unrealistic expectations from above and below. My admonition to my colleagues is to respond with measured words, grace, and empathy no matter how hard it is to be civil. In the end you are first and foremost a physician.

                                   CHRISTOPHER C. COLENDA, MD, MPH
                                   DEAN, TEXAS A&M COLLEGE OF MEDICINE

- **When dealing with difficult people, sometimes take the opposite approach.**

Most of our colleagues are friendly and rational. Unfortunately, this is not true of all of them. When you are confronted with people who are hostile, aggressive, sarcastic, or negative, listen carefully, try to understand their position, and "kill them with kindness." They will usually calm down so that you can converse or negotiate with them effectively. A counterattack is rarely but occasionally necessary, and it can also be effective. Dealing with whiners and overly pleasant or agreeable people often takes a more direct approach. If reaching an agreement continues to be difficult, it may be time to delegate this function to someone else who can arbitrate.

> Do you have the courage to kill your own snakes?

- **Become involved in succession planning.**

One important function of leaders is to train others to replace them. This involves helping others develop self-awareness, monitoring their progress and providing feedback, letting people know what they are doing wrong so that they can improve, removing obstacles to their progress, and teaching them. To this extent, the learner is usually reluctant to approach you; you must approach the learner.

- **Have a plan for terminating others. Here are some approaches.**

I have found it is difficult to have chairs step down even though they know it's time. With no strict retirement ages at Hopkins, I needed to devise a way to make this happen without much fuss. One of the most effective ways is to call in a chair, discuss how his/her department is going, and then say, "Who do you think should be the chair of your search committee?" After the mouth has closed, he/she has to respond with some names. There is no time for discussion, so you move on.

EDWARD D. MILLER MD
DEAN, JOHNS HOPKINS SCHOOL OF MEDICINE

The hardest conversation that a dean has with a chair is the last one, when it is time for the chair to move on. There are many ways to begin, talking about succession, the lure of a fishing line, or the various issues that have probably been rehashed several times in the past. However, I really think that the dean should not feel as though it is necessary to make excuses for what is best for the institution. So, I simply start by saying, "I've made a decision. We are going to make a change in the leadership of your department. The decision is already made now, so we don't need to spend any time arguing about whether it is right or wrong. Let's concentrate on how you are going to move on, what we are both going to say, and what the best approach for the department is going to be during the transition."

THOMAS A. DEUTSCH, MD
DEAN, RUSH MEDICAL SCHOOL

Most subordinates have no clue that they are not effective, or if they do, won't admit it. Be careful not to personalize the issue. Asking a chair or key administrator or even a faculty member to step down is not only threatening to that person but to all others in similar positions. The first thing to do when you are planning to terminate someone is to clear it with your superiors, all the way to the president, and occasionally the president may want to notify or consult with the trustees. What the person terminated will want to do is to test your decision with your superior. Try to create a way for them to save face in the process. One possibility would be to meet with the person, tell him his strengths and weaknesses, and then say that you are going to schedule a meeting three days later during which you will ask him to step down. In the interim, he should think of "comfortable" ways this can happen: announce his stepping down in three months because of fatigue, looking for other opportunities, etc. Be prepared for a negative reaction. When a person has been terminated, there is an irresistible urge to talk to someone (faculty, friends, your superiors, etc.) in the hope that he can reverse the decision. Once you have made a decision to terminate, negotiate only when, not whether.

• **There may be times when shame is an effective weapon.**
It is not uncommon to hear from faculty members that they don't have time to teach or that they are not paid to teach. Without doubt, we clearly expect more now from the faculty in research and clinical productivity, but teaching the next generations of health professionals is not only an obligation of the faculty but also a duty. A reminder of the Hippocratic oath and its contract between teachers and students may be appropriate at this point.

• **For projects that require input from faculty members, provide something in writing to which they can respond.**
There is nothing worse that writing a mission and vision statement by committee. Everyone wants to be a wordsmith. In a situation like this, consider writing a statement and asking the others to respond to it. It may also be good to allow the group members to free-associate on an idea and then return to them later with something more specific in writing to which they can respond.

> It's amazing how much easier it is for a team to work together when no one has the slightest idea where they are going.

• **While raising three boys, my wife and I made the following observation.**
When someone did something nice for the two of us, it most likely generated a thank you note, but if some act of kindness or something with special significance was given to our boys, we as parents became forever grateful. It is with this "pearl" that my wife and I decided to purchase sterling silver baby cups for each medical student who has a baby during medical school. The cup, engraved with the baby's name, birth date, parent's name, and the school's name, is presented to the baby and parents at a brief dedication ceremony in front of the medical school class. We do this to emphasize the importance of family and to give the family a lasting memento from the school that helps them remember their school with fondness.

H. ROGER HADLEY, MD
DEAN, LOMA LINDA SCHOOL OF MEDICINE

• **You can't understand everyone's motives.**
If you don't understand someone's behavior, you don't have enough history.

RICHARD D. KRUGMAN, MD
DEAN, UNIVERSITY OF COLORADO SCHOOL OF MEDICINE

> A dean and a medical student were walking along when they came upon a small frog on the sidewalk. The frog said to the dean, "If you will pick me up and kiss me, I will turn into a beautiful young woman," The dean picked the frog up and put it in his pocket. When the student questioned why he didn't kiss the frog, the dean said, "At my age, I'd rather have a talking frog."

CHAPTER 12

Relating to the Media

For many academic leaders, relating to the media can be a new and sometimes daunting experience. Most institutions have a public relations staff that organizes and manages public appearances and media interactions. Individual faculty members are involved only when their expertise is needed. Institutional leaders, however, are expected to be knowledgeable about most if not all of the school's programs and to be able to communicate with the school's constituents as needed.

Use interactions with the media as opportunities to promote your institution or academic unit. Many new administrators have never had the experience of interacting with the media. Most reporters are pleasant and accommodating. They are only interested in getting information about a particular topic so that they can meet a deadline, whether it is in the print or electronic media. In most communities, the reporters certainly don't want to alienate you because they know that they may want more information later on the same or another subject and that they will need your cooperation. Rarely will you encounter an investigative reporter, one who is looking for specific information about a sensitive or legal issue. In the latter situation, you are more likely to be "ambushed" with difficult questions during a press conference or walking from one location to another. Fortunately, this seldom happens. But remember, the media will tell the story with or without you, and the story without you is less likely to include your key messages. The following are pearls that may be helpful when interacting with the media and others outside the institution. By the way, don't expect reporters to compliment you on your response to their questions. Most of the time, they are interested only in your saying something for the record, not necessarily what you said or how you said it.

- **Use every opportunity to talk to the public about the school, faculty, and students.**

A message usually needs to be heard three times before it is retained. The public is bombarded with messages from other hospitals, schools, and institutions. It is important to take the opportunity to remind the public of your school's mission several times before it is retained. It is also crucial that you relate the message to the public in a way for them to care. For instance, talking about improving the educational curriculum of the school is one thing, but talking about developing a new curriculum to develop better physicians who will be more sensitive to their patients and their needs relates more to the public and what they will get out of your mission. Help them understand why they should care.

> Things are more like they are now than they have ever been before.

- **Be prepared to "say something"—anytime, anywhere.**
You will often be asked to talk on an impromptu basis. It can happen at any time and when you are totally unprepared. If you say you don't want to talk, you look as if you are ignorant of the topic. If you don't know what to say, you prove it. When unprepared, think of the three missions—education, research, and service—to organize your thoughts. Usually the subject of the meeting, no matter what it is, will fit into one or more of these missions and you can structure your impromptu comments around the missions and your goals. You should be able to recite in your sleep the goal you have for each of these missions.

- **Dress appropriately for the interview.**
Solid white shirts and suits with plaid patterns or stripes do not show well on camera or in a photograph. Wear solid-color shirts and solid-color suits. Men should also avoid busy ties on camera. Whether you like it or not, how you appear on camera or in a photograph is how the public will judge you. A warm day creating perspiration on your brow can make you appear guilty on camera. Always take a few minutes and make sure you are put together before looking into the lens.

- **When on camera, talk to the interviewer.**
Don't talk to the camera. Just engage in a conversation with the interviewer. Don't be a "doctor" when talking to the media; they will want everything in layman's terms. Don't touch your face with your hands because, on camera, it always looks like you are going for your nose.

- **Nothing is ever "off the record."**
Some reporters will try to get you to just have a conversation with them off the record. This is never the case. Anything you say to a reporter can be used. So, always keep your guard up and only say things that wouldn't give you heartburn if you saw them in print the next day.

- **Take advantage of every interaction with the media.**
Think about the one or two things you want to get across in a statement or sound bite and work them into the conversation. No matter what the question is, always try to bridge back to the key messages when possible. Your sound bite will be only a few seconds, so keep your comments brief and to the point. The more interesting you make the comment, the more likely the reporter will quote you in the story.

> To paraphrase Mr. Lincoln, you can fool some of the people all of the time and all of the people some of the time, and sometimes that's enough.

- **Don't talk to fill the silence.**
Some reporters like to leave silence in hopes you'll begin talking again. Inevitably when you do, you begin to talk about things that are off the key message or

say things that lead to other questions that you'd rather not talk about. Answer the reporter's question in a sound bite and then just wait for the next question. Don't fill the silence.

> Listening never gets you into trouble. Talking can.

- **Know the reporter.**
Your public relations office should provide you with some history on the reporter before the interview. If not, request it. It's important to know what types of stories the reporter normally covers so that you can relate to them. If they typically find the negative side of any story, you need to know that to be better prepared. If they've never covered health care or research, you can brief them on the significance behind certain points. Otherwise, the story will not be on target.

- **When a VIP is in the hospital or there is some major media event, the media can be very demanding of your time.**
Establish a time and place where you or someone will meet with the press on a regular basis. Consult with your public relations department. They should manage all of the logistics for you, including the media's requests.

- **Be aware of the media "mole."**
There will always be a staff or faculty member who will notify the press of something of interest, so be prepared to have to address the media about it. Compromising information in particular is seldom a secret.

- **Notify your superiors of any event that may reach the media so they won't be surprised.**
If you ever wonder whether you should tell your superiors about an issue or event that may be important or especially something that may be embarrassing to the institution, tell them. That's better than their finding out about it and asking why you didn't tell them.

- **Be proactive and open about errors and communicate a plan to resolve them.**
If there is a major blunder, it is better to be proactive and go public with it than to have investigative reporters get involved. The issue does not become news if you openly address it before others find out about it. Otherwise it becomes a series of negative media reports that are bad for the institution and for you. If you don't know all of the details about the event, be honest. Meet with the reporters on a regular basis until the negative issue is resolved. Let the media know what you know and what you are still working on to resolve the issue. Be quick to respond to the media's requests. If you delay and they are scheduled to produce a story, they will find out on their own without your influence on the message, many times telling an angle that could have been avoided if you worked with them from the beginning. Don't forget to keep the faculty and staff up to date on the situation as well. The last thing you want is for your employees to have to learn about the situation from the media. They should hear it directly from you to make sure they get the correct information.

- **Don't repeat the reporter's negative comments.**

If you are asked a negative question, don't repeat it in your response. If you do, that will be the sound bite the reporter uses in the story. Just comment on the positive things you are going to do to fix the situation.

- **Have the media and all media questions routed through a public affairs office.**

Administrators have a tendency to want to talk to the media about positive things but refer the negative issues to the public affairs staff. Always have the media first contact a public affairs person about a story rather than talking to you. The public affairs staff person can determine what the issue is about and talk to you before you have to talk to the media. That gives you time to think about what you will say.

- **Always have a public relations representative present during an interview.**

While it is good for the public relations office to know all of the messages that are being disseminated to the press, this item is more important for you than anyone. If you are misquoted by the press, you have no one to back you up unless the PR person from your institution is present.

- **Don't put anything on paper unless you are prepared to see it in the media.**

Be careful what you write in a letter or a report because you may see it again … on the front page of the paper or on television. The same is true for electronic mail. Anything written can come back to haunt you. Never write anything when you are angry. If you do write a scathing letter, put it in a drawer for a day or two before sending it. When you settle down, you may be glad you didn't send it.

- **It is OK to say, "I don't know."**

If you don't know the answer to a question, don't make up or guess the answer. Have you ever heard anyone saying, "I don't know" quoted in the newspaper or on television? Never! Just tell the reporter you don't know the answer. If it is important, you can offer to provide the information later.

> Before I heard your lecture, I was confused. I am still confused but on a much higher level. – Enrico Fermi to J. Robert Oppenheimer

CHAPTER 13

Connecting to the Community

The intensity of the education of the medical scientist and academic clinician is well known. Once we complete training, our work revolves around promotions and tenure, often to the neglect of family and friends. Success frequently depends on our prominence in national conferences and specialty societies. Often, the norm is to have several moves to institutions in different cities. As administrators, we find comfort in adding new obligations to organizations like the Association of American Medical Colleges, which have further impact on a tight schedule. Few take the time to think of their responsibilities to the community in which they live and work. The community, in this respect, can take the form of organized medicine or local service organizations.

From the community's perspective, the people believe that they are supporting the school, whether it is private or public. They want to know and be involved with the school leaders on a personal basis. To ignore their desires is to court failure as an administrator, particularly if there is a crisis in the school when community support is needed. Medical school leaders at all levels of administration should become involved with community interests. The following pearls relate to community involvement.

- **Your image in the community is important.**
A major academic administrative position is time-consuming within the organization. Yet, your image in the community can be all-important in fund raising, in relating to the legislators and other political offices, and in keeping a positive public image for the institution. Service on selected boards and visibly supporting some charitable institutions are essential to maintaining a positive community image.

> Do what you ought to do when you ought to do it whether you want to do it or not.

- **Have a good administrative assistant.**
How your administrative assistant relates to faculty, alumni, VIPs, and others on the phone and in the office is a reflection on you and the whole school.

- **Identify those for whom you should be interrupted.**
Your administrative assistant should know that there are some people—the governor, alumni, referring physicians, certain others—whom you should talk to when they call and, unless you are in an important meeting, you should be interrupted to take the call.

- **Determine how much time can be allocated to the community.**

Time management is the key. Decide how much time is necessary for academic and family work, and set aside a certain amount of time for community issues. Such activities may coincide with academic interests, personal interests, or school priorities.

- **Determine whether to focus service on organized medicine or on community service agencies and organizations.**

As an academic leader, active involvement in organized medicine is expected. This involvement should be, to some extent, at the local, state, and national levels even if involvement means only membership and participation. Community involvement at the local service organization level should focus on how to relate to political and business leaders of the community or state. Service organizations such as the Rotary Club or Chamber of Commerce or agencies that support the arts are good places to start. It is helpful to have a spouse to share some of these activities. Your involvement should be in something for which you have passion and not be purely for social climbing or self-interest.

- **Establish a relationship with the local media.**

Don't overlook the power of the publisher and editor of a local newspaper or the electronic media. True friendships with opinion leaders can be important to solving problems and gaining public support before there is a crisis.

> One can never have too many friends, but one enemy is too many.

- **Be generous with your contributions to worthy causes.**

If you expect the community to be generous in support of your institution, find ways to give back to the community, whether in time or money. Your success as an academic administrator may be more closely tied to your relationship with community leaders than your excellence as a scientist and physician.

- **Cultivate friends from different backgrounds.**

Use community relationships to develop friendships of varying backgrounds in order to broaden your understanding of the community and to gain a better understanding of the importance of the role of your institution in it. This allows the opportunity to gain different perspectives of what people think of the school and what it is doing for the community.

- **Plan the approach to fund-raising carefully.**

The ideal way to approach a donor is with a member of the board of trustees and an involved faculty member. The selection of each is critical and must be carefully done. Of primary importance is the trustee's own example of giving. People who are the most successful in raising money are those who give money. It's hard to convince someone else to give to a worthy cause if the solicitor is not also contributing. Do not make the pitch until you have an idea of an area of interest of the potential donor. The specifics should give enough leeway to try to accommodate the interests of all involved. Always have a backup plan. Few people are insulted by overshooting the ask target. They will never claim to be insulted by asking them for too little, but you will shortchange your own fund-raising efforts by doing so. Finally, have a strategic plan tied closely to the fund-raising and stick to it. Each donor's situation is different and each carries its own unique set of requirements.

Antonio M. Gotto, MD
Dean, Cornell Weill Medical College

- **Consider having advisory boards for community and alumni relations.**

Some schools have separate boards of trustees or regents that serve as advisory groups. If you don't have a separate board, a group of community or national advisors can be very valuable, and they can also make significant monetary or other contributions to the school.

A dean claimed that he once met the queen of England. At least, that is what she said. She said, "If you are the dean of a medical school, I must be the queen of England."

CHAPTER 14

Talking About Things We Don't Like to Talk About

No one wants to have to leave a leadership position. Consequently, leaders often remain in a position longer than they should. Sometimes they don't detect the warning signs that they should step down, and sometimes they just ignore them. If a leader steps down too early, he/she is disappointed, and if the leader waits too long to resign, everyone else is disappointed. It helps to have negotiated an exit strategy when accepting the leadership position (see Chapter 2).

> One should not look back in anger nor forward in fear, but around with awareness. – Senator Nancy Kassebaum

- **You should step down from your position when…**
  …it's no longer fun.
  …you try to avoid confrontation.
  …it becomes important to be popular.
  …you are concerned about what you would do if you weren't in the job.
  …you are persistently angry at the "administration" or others.
  …there is consistent lack of support from superiors.
  …you no longer are able to get the resources you need to run the unit.
  …your immediate superior tells you to, or hints strongly.

> Life is a dash between two numbers on a tombstone. Enjoy it.

- **When others stop listening, start looking.**
Deans, chairs, and other administrators seem to be more effective and seem to accomplish more in the early years of their tenure, and they often lose effectiveness after ten to twelve years because they no longer have good ideas, they lose their passion for the work, or no one listens to them. This is another way of saying that they can no longer obtain the financial resources to initiate and implement new programs. A few people continue to be effective, but only in exceptional circumstances should they continue in the same position beyond ten to twelve years. Instead, they should look for another position or another institution. This is one more reason for negotiating the divorce when you negotiate the marriage (see Chapter 2).

- **Plan your exit.**

There is a time in life for everything. Leave while they still want you. If they're glad to see you go, you've stayed too long.

Lewis Landsberg, MD
Dean, Northwestern University
Feinberg School of Medicine

- **There is life after administration. More administration.**

Many administrators who leave a position find themselves in other administrative positions. Some move up the administrative ladder to associate dean, dean, or vice president. Some have even become university presidents. Some have moved to government positions.

> When you foster anger, you only allow someone to continue to hurt you.

- **Every medical school needs interim leadership.**

Every medical school has dean, associate dean, chair, or center director positions that are open from time to time. A good administrator could fill any of these positions on an interim basis. Dr. James Glenn, who was dean at Emory University School of Medicine and president of Mt. Sinai Hospital, served in several interim positions—chair of surgery, associate dean for clinical affairs, director of the cancer center—upon his return to the University of Kentucky. There should be a consulting company called "Interim, Inc.," a company that would provide interim leadership for medical schools across the country. There are plenty of former medical school administrators who could fill the interim roles.

> If you can't think what you would do after being in a leadership position, you shouldn't have been in the position in the first place.

- **Health policy in the United States needs your help.**

Because of their experience in medical administration, many former administrators become involved in health policy at the state or national levels.

- **Consider working with national organizations.**

National health care organizations and specialty organizations need experienced administrators. Dr. John Clarkson, former dean at the University of Miami School of Medicine, became the executive director of the American Board of Ophthalmology.

- **Consult a headhunter.**

Several search firms now consult with medical schools to find capable leaders for various positions throughout the hierarchy. Some former medical school administrators now serve as consultants for these companies. Contact these companies to see what opportunities are available.

- **Acknowledge that administration may not be your strength.**

Administration is not for everyone. Sometimes it is better to just acknowledge that and return to doing what you do best—teaching or research or service. Sir William Osler wanted his epitaph to read, "I taught medical students." There is no finer task.

The best known joke about deans is the one about the "three letters." As the story goes, a new dean was being oriented to his office when the retiring dean told him that if he ever had a problem, he should consult the advice in one of the three letters he had prepared and left in his desk. Things went well for a while but before long the new dean developed a major problem with the faculty. Remembering his predecessor's advice, he opened the first letter in his desk which said, "Blame your predecessor." This he did and things seemed to go well for a while until a second problem arose. The new dean consulted the second letter which said, "Blame the university president." Again, things began to improve only to turn worse later with another problem. He then opened the third letter which said, "Prepare three letters." Perhaps the following algorithm can help with decision-making.

Algorithm for Academic Problem Solving

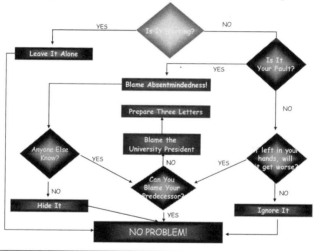

CHAPTER 15

Applying Management Principles to Academic Leadership

Medical schools, with their escalating clinical and research programs, function a lot like major corporations but they must do so in an academic environment. Unlike corporations, universities have a structured hierarchy and volumes of regulations to compensate for a lack of discipline among the faculty or, in rare cases, incompetence. Academic freedom is a virtue, but it is by definition antithetical to the corporate discipline necessary to focus attention and resources on selected components of the mission. Instead, faculty members are free to pursue any interest, and medical schools often promote mediocrity by spreading resources equitably across numerous programs. Lack of discipline is prevalent in all sectors of a university as demonstrated by lack of research focus, failure to meet grant deadlines, being late to clinic, and not communicating with referring physicians.

It is possible for academic institutions to correct these problems, but it requires knowledge of business principles and a culture of discipline. To balance the corporate nature of medical schools with the academic missions and to improve system efficiency and effectiveness, administrators have begun to apply business principles to medical school operations.

The principles outlined as success factors for companies are basic premises that can improve the operations of a medical school if they are incorporated into its culture. The pearls in this chapter are case studies that demonstrate how business principles can be used in an academic setting.

- **First Who, Then What**

The good-to-great leaders began the transformation by first getting the right people on the bus (and the wrong people off the bus) and then figured out where to drive it … "who" questions come before "what" questions. … We uncovered three practical disciplines for being rigorous in people decisions:

1. When in doubt, don't hire—keep looking.
2. When you know you need to make a people change, act.
3. Put your best people on your biggest opportunities, not your biggest problems.

JIM COLLINS
GOOD TO GREAT

Getting the right people on the bus and the wrong people off the bus can be difficult in an academic setting. Academic freedom, tenure, and other academic conventions often interfere with what might otherwise be good personnel decisions.

For example, should a new leader request the resignations of all direct reports in order to build a more cohesive team, or should the new leader evaluate the current administrators for six months or so before selecting permanent team members? Unfortunately, there is no clear-cut answer to this question. On two occasions, one of the authors declined to bring in new people at the outset even though he was convinced they had better skill sets to be effective and to fit his management style. In both cases, he found it just as painful, if not more so, to make administrative changes months later. In contrast, on another occasion, he decided not to make major staff changes despite encouragement from organizational leadership, and the outcome turned out to be excellent. A new leader should meet with direct reports frequently and early in one's tenure to determine if they have the personal and management skills compatible with the anticipated changes in the organization. If not, they should be replaced with the "right people on the bus" in a timely manner. Of more importance is to make personnel changes over a short timeframe whether the changes occur early or later in one's tenure, and not string out the dismissals over several months, which only creates undue stress among the administrative team.

- **Begin with the End in Mind**
To begin with the end in mind means to start with a clear understanding of your destination. It means to know where you're going so that you better understand where you are now and so that the steps you take are always in the right direction.

STEPHEN R. COVEY
THE 7 HABITS OF HIGHLY EFFECTIVE PEOPLE

Every organization needs leaders and followers. The leader must create clear goals and then be allowed to be creative, to take risks, and to make mistakes in order to meet those goals. The successes we admire today are because of leaders who could "think big" and who had the capacity to dream and who then had the energy and wherewithal to carry it out.

I found that if an idea would "work" in my mind, if I could visualize the end in mind, then the idea could be accomplished. If I couldn't create and bring about a project in my mind, then I was reluctant to support it until I had more information and could envision it.

Kentucky Governor A.B. "Happy" Chandler and founding dean William Willard had a dream of a second medical school in Kentucky when others said it wasn't needed or that it couldn't be done. That dream led to the University of Kentucky College of Medicine. Another example occurred when President Charles Odegaard established the University of Washington, only the second medical school in the entire northwest United States, as one of the nation's most prominent schools in education, research and clinical care.

> To make a great dream come true, the first requirement is a capacity to dream. The second is persistence of faith in the dream.
>
> Hans Selye
>
> It doesn't matter what you think or what I think. When history is written, it will be what you do and what I do.
>
> Governor A.B. "Happy" Chandler

- ## You Can Choose to Have a Good Day

As you enter this place of work please choose to make today a great day. Your colleagues, customers, team members, and you yourself will be thankful. Find ways to play. We can be serious about our work without being serious about ourselves. Stay focused in order to be present when your customers and team members most need you. And should you feel your energy lapsing, try this surefire remedy: Find someone who needs a helping hand, a word of support, or a good ear—and make their day.

Stephen C. Lundin, Harry Paul, and John Christensen
Fish !

I was having a bad day, to say the least. Then, I was called to the office of the university president one afternoon at four o'clock. I did not know the reason for the meeting, but the day before I had given a presentation to an architectural committee, arguing for a new building to be located adjacent to the medical school. The meeting was short. The president told me that if I didn't wish to have the building where he wanted it, I could resign. The meeting lasted three minutes. When I left the office, I was both somewhat confused and angry. I didn't know what to do. I never meant my position to be an affront to the president. I was only stating an opinion. My first impulse was to return to my office and talk to my colleagues about what I had just experienced.

When we have an unpleasant experience, we often have an irresistible urge to tell someone. We want their support and their sympathy. I now understood why those I had terminated in the past did just that. However, a meeting with the president was a private meeting, and if others somehow found out what had been said (which is exactly what happened), I didn't want the president to think that I was the one who told anyone.

Instead, I went to work the next morning and called in a new colleague who had been with the university only two weeks and said, "Your predecessor was here for thirteen years and during that time, my job was never threatened. I am going to give you two more weeks and if you can't get me fired by then, we will have to talk again."

- ## Selecting an Administrative Team

Who you are today is a result of certain characteristics that have emerged from your life experiences, plus the genetics with which you were born. This interplay between nature and nurture is the foundation ... of a brain-based approach to personality profiling that gives you the keys you need to discover not only your strengths and talents but also those of others.

Steven Geil Browning
Emergenetics

As a dean, I was always looking for ways to improve the management skills of associate deans, chairs, and other administrators. I used speakers, consultants, and oftentimes concepts from the world of business. We have all submitted to personality profiles such as the Myers-Briggs Profile, so I involved the administrators in a process called Emergenetics (www.emergenetics.com/emergenetics/masterpages/default.aspx), which "helps ... build stronger, more creative and productive teams." Using a questionnaire, it categorizes an individual into one of four groups: analytical, structural, social, and conceptual. Some administrators were clearly in one group while others were mixtures of two profiles. I prefer to think of the profiles as follows:

1. Detail oriented: those who can't get enough facts. They often can't make a decision because they don't have enough information. They know how much money they have in the bank—to the penny.
2. Organized: those who are very structured in their lives. They like to put things in boxes, like an organization chart. They know how much money they have in the bank within a few dollars.
3. Considerate: those who are very considerate of others. When a subject is being discussed, their first question is, "Yes, but how will this affect this other person or group?" They have no idea how much money is in their bank account.
4. Visionary: those who are always in the clouds, constantly coming up with great ideas, some of which are practical and some not. They don't know if they even have a bank account.

To be an effective organization, we need all of these personality types on our team. If the team consisted only of the detail-oriented or of visionaries, we could never accomplish anything because we could never get enough information in the one case or we would never face reality in the other. We need to acknowledge the importance of different administrative and personality profiles.

- **Invent Options for Mutual Gain**
  To invent creative options, then, you will need (1) to separate the act of inventing options from the act of judging them, (2) to broaden the options on the table rather than look for a single answer, (3) to search for mutual gains, and (4) to invent ways of making decisions easy.
  ROGER FISHER AND WILLIAM URY
GETTING TO YES: NEGOTIATING AGREEMENT WITHOUT GIVING IN

Young faculty members, and older ones as well, are often like children. Once they have been appointed and provided with space, equipment, and other institutional possessions, it is "Mine! Mine! Mine!" I must admit that when I first became a faculty member, I had the same attitude. I was given two laboratories, an office, and major pieces of equipment to start my research program. Singular ownership of research resources in particular was important to me.

At the beginning of my second year on the faculty, I heard that another faculty member had received a grant and that he would need laboratory space. I knew that all of the other laboratories assigned to the department were fully utilized and, since I did not yet have a grant, I "judged" that one of my laboratories would be reassigned to someone else.

Mustering all my courage, I marched into the department chair's office and indicated to him that I was concerned about a schism in the department if this happened. He listened patiently, discussed other options including the sharing of space and equipment, and left me with the impression that he indeed understood the problem and that he would give it serious thought.

A week later, to my surprise, I learned that the chair had obtained an additional laboratory from the medical school administration and that I would be allowed to keep my laboratories as promised in my letter of appointment. It turned out to be a win-win situation and a mutual gain for the other faculty member and me.

• Creating a Succession Plan

Succession planning and management is the process that helps ensure the stability of the tenure of personnel. It is perhaps best understood as any effort designed to ensure the continued effective performance of an organization by making provision for the development, replacement, and strategic application of key people over time.

WILLIAM J. ROTHWELL
EFFECTIVE SUCCESSION PLANNING

Leading an academic medical school is difficult, in part because of participatory governance and the need to involve faculty members in every major decision. Nowhere is this problem more prevalent than in the search process and succession planning. The selection of university administrators is at best a cumbersome if not flawed process. Good candidates from within the university are often overlooked in favor of outside candidates who are perceived to bring new ideas to the institution. Being an outstanding educator or researcher does not necessarily equate with being a charismatic leader or manager. When searching for an administrator, I always tried to keep in mind the "recruiting commandments" proposed by Dr. R. G. Petersdorf, former president of the Association of American Medical Colleges:

1. Thou shalt keep search committees small.
2. Thou shalt encourage advertising for all jobs.
3. Thou shalt not harass your colleagues with needless letters.
4. Thou shalt set a time limit on the duration of the search process.
5. Thou shalt obtain data selectively and not canvass the universe.
6. Thou shalt keep candidates' visits humanely short.
7. Thou shalt avoid committee deadlocks.
8. Thou shalt shun faculty stew.
9. Thou shalt feel free to search without a committee.
10. Thou shalt not ignore excellent inside candidates.

Succession planning and the search process are probably the weakest elements in our ability to build a strong medical school. Because of the expense of the search process in time, money, and people, and because great leaders can come from within, medical schools should put more emphasis on succession planning at all administrative levels.

• Managing by Walking Around

Catching people doing things right is a powerful management concept. Unfortunately, most leaders have a genius for catching people doing things wrong. I always recommend that leaders spend at least an hour a week wandering around their operation catching people doing things right.

KENNETH BLANCHARD AND SPENCER JOHNSON
THE ONE MINUTE MANAGER

As a senior administrator, it was difficult for me to communicate with the faculty except by faculty meetings, newsletters, or the occasional random conversation. I never felt that I knew very much about what was really going on in my institution or what people were thinking or were concerned about. Even though I had an open-door policy, it just didn't work very well. Those who took advantage of it were the more vocal or disgruntled ones. The others never came in. I could not always depend on the associate deans or chairs because even if they knew of faculty concerns, they often did not want to upset me with bad news.

I finally decided that if I really wanted to know what the faculty was thinking, I needed to schedule time on my calendar to find out. I scheduled time each day to walk through different areas of my responsibility to talk to members of the faculty and staff. I always went by myself, and I walked the hallways and into laboratories, offices, and clinics. In the hospital, I even made an effort to schedule time to meet the staff on different shifts. I smiled a lot and tried to make myself available for people to talk with me in an unthreatening environment. It was my attempt to manage by walking around. I was surprised at what I could learn, and I was even more surprised by the accolades I received for just being friendly and available. I also learned a lot by watching their facial expressions and their body language. In the words of Yogi Berra, "You can observe a lot just by watching."

In addition to gaining information, I found that I actually enjoyed this time with the faculty, staff, and students. And it's nice to get out of the office from time to time and just have fun!

- **Seek First to Understand, Then to Be Understood**

Listen empathetically, seek to understand both what is said and the emotion behind it, diagnose before prescribing, then communicate demonstrating credibility, empathy and logic.

STEPHEN R. COVEY
THE 7 HABITS OF HIGHLY EFFECTIVE PEOPLE

When you find yourself dealing with someone who is stubborn, disruptive, disrespectful, or belligerent, you must first be patient and listen to the conversation. Remember that, for the most part, everyone wants to be loved, appreciated, and respected. Before responding, try to "get into the other person's head." What is he or she really trying to say and why? Once you have a good understanding of his or her position, you can begin to address the problem.

Maybe you aren't presenting your position in a manner that others can understand. If faculty members are not part of the discussions leading up to the point of your decision, they don't know the history and may not fully understand your position. Try a different approach in order to gain more understanding. If the person confronting you is still problematic, ask the person to come to your office to discuss the situation further in private.

It seems that every faculty group has its self-designated adversary, some of whom are well meaning but most of whom are antagonistic toward administrators in particular. The rest of the faculty members often depend on this individual to express what they are thinking but are afraid to say. This person is usually the first person to ask a question after your presentation, often to the smiles of the rest of the group. When you become aware of this pattern, you can often defuse the situation by actually calling on this person at the conclusion of your remarks with something like, "Well, Mike, I'm sure you have a question."

Whatever the level of confrontation, never, never, never get angry. Smile and be your diplomatic self.

References and Selected Readings

References

Blanchard, K.H., and Johnson, S.: *The One Minute Manager,* William Morrow and Company, New York, 1982.

Browning, G.: *Emergenetics,* HarperCollins Publishers, New York, 2006.

Clawson, D.K., and Wilson, E.A.: *The Medical School Dean: Reflections and Directions,* McClanahan Publishing House, Katawa, Kentucky, 1999.

Collins, J.: *Good to Great,* HarperCollins Publishers, New York, 2001.

Collins, J.C., and Porras, J.I.: *Built to Last,* HarperCollins Publishers, New York, 1997.

Covey, S.R.: *The 7 Habits of Highly Effective People,* Fireside, Simon & Schuster, Inc., New York, 1990.

Fisher, R., and Ury, W.: *Getting to Yes: Negotiating Agreement Without Giving In,* Penguin Books, New York, 1981.

Lundin, S.C., Paul, H., and Christensen, J.: *Fish!,* Hyperion, New York, 1996.

Machiavelli, N.: *The Prince,* Penguin Books, New York, 1988.

Rothwell, W.J.: *Effective Succession Planning: Insuring Leadership Continuity and Building Talent from Within,* AMACOM, New York, 2005.

Shapiro, R.M., and Jankowski, M.A.: *The Power of Nice: How to Negotiate So Everyone Wins,* John Wiley and Sons, Inc., New York, 1998, 2001.

Thaler, L.K., and Koval, R.: *The Power of Nice: How to Conquer the Business World with Kindness,* Doubleday, New York, 2006.

Selected Readings

Blanchard, K., and Lorber, R.: *Putting the One Minute Manager to Work,* William Morrow and Company, New York, 1984.

Gladwell, M.: *Blink,* Little, Brown and Company, New York, 2005.

Gladwell, M.: *The Tipping Point,* Little, Brown and Company, New York, 2000.

Johnson, S.: *Who Moved My Cheese?* G.P. Putnam's Sons, New York, 1999.

Thomas, J.: *Negotiate to Win,* HarperCollins Publishers, New York, 2005.

Index

—

Printed in the United States